The Vitality Mark

Dr Mark Rowe has been a practising family physician for over 25 years and is a thought leader in the areas of positive health and lifestyle medicine. In 2008, he founded the Waterford Health Park, where his medical practice and 'be well suite' is located. The innovative site espouses Dr Rowe's core values in terms of primary healthcare provision and received a global health improvement award in 2013.

After his own experience of burnout, Dr Rowe became one of the first medical doctors in Ireland to study lifestyle medicine, and his passion for wellbeing has since led to his being certified as a diplomate of the International Board of Lifestyle Medicine, as well as being appointed an honorary senior lecturer at the RCSI School of Medicine and Health Sciences. As a keynote speaker, Dr Rowe has delivered events and workshops all over the world, and his 2017 TEDx Talk was titled 'The Doctor of the Future: Prescribing Lifestyle as Medicine'. He has written previous books including *A Prescription for Happiness: Ten Commitments for a Happier, Healthier Life* and *The Men's Health Book*, and also hosts the wellbeing podcast *In the Doctor's Chair*.

For resources and to learn more about Dr Rowe and his work, please visit drmarkrowe.com.

The Vitality Mark

Your prescription for feeling
energised, invigorated,
enthusiastic and optimistic
each day

Dr Mark Rowe

Gill Books

Gill Books
Hume Avenue
Park West
Dublin 12
www.gillbooks.ie

Gill Books is an imprint of M.H. Gill and Co.

978 07171 9280 9

Design and print origination by O'K Graphic Design, Dublin
Edited by Sheila Armstrong
Illustration by Derry Dillon
Printed by CPI Group (UK) Ltd, Croydon, CR0 4YY

This book is typeset in Minion Pro 11/17 pt

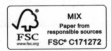

A CIP catalogue record for this book is available from the British Library.

5 4 3 2 1

Foreword

I first met Dr Mark Rowe in person in 2017, when I was presenting a lecture on behaviour change for a Harvard Medical School CME (continuing medical education) course that he attended – and we've kept in contact digitally ever since. I've been able to follow Dr Rowe's wisdom and insights through social media, videos and his podcast, *In the Doctor's Chair*. This book now compiles his thoughts and theories into one easy-to-read resource; and, given the Covid-19 pandemic, the timing for *The Vitality Mark* could not be better, as people are struggling to find new ways to connect, to use stress-reduction techniques, to eat a healthy diet that can help our immune systems to best function and to set ourselves up for sound sleep at night.

How we move our bodies, what foods we enjoy, how many hours we sleep, how we handle stressful situations and our dedication to building high-quality connections all have an impact on our sense of wellbeing. Hippocrates spoke centuries ago about the first two of these important factors, and has been credited with saying 'Walking is man's best medicine' and 'If we could give every individual the right amount of nourishment and exercise, not too little and not too much, we would have found the safest way to health'.

More and more research supports these statements. Studies from the past couple of decades demonstrate how sleep impacts our bodies and brains, and how we suffer without sleep. It impacts many different areas of our lives and organs in our bodies, from the amount of food we crave and consume to the level of ghrelin (a hormone that increases our appetite) in our system. Psychiatrists and cardiologists have also been interested in the impact stress can have on the heart since at least 1988, when Alan Rozanski and colleagues demonstrated that mental stress could impact wall motion of the heart and myocardial ischemia. In fact, this research led me to study the impact of mental stress – specifically serial subtraction by seven, a test frequently used in dementia evaluations – on the heart–wall motion as well as EKG readings.

Our social connections also have a profound effect on our lives at every age. It was my own father's heart attack and stroke, which he suffered at age 52, that put me on the path to medical school, and I have since gone on to further explore the prevention and treatment of heart attacks and strokes. The Covid-19 pandemic has brought the power of high-quality connections to the forefront of medicine and made it a priority for most people around the world. The six pillars of lifestyle medicine (exercise, healthy eating, sleep, stress resilience, social connection and avoidance of risky substances) all help to keep us healthy and add to our sense of wellbeing.

Vitality is defined by the Merriam Webster Dictionary as, firstly, 'a lively or energetic quality' and, secondly, 'the power or ability of something to continue to live, be successful'. Vitality is wellbeing and more. By paying attention to our body, mind, heart and soul, we can increase our feeling of vitality – as Dr Rowe explains in this book. *The Vitality Mark* invites the reader to embark on a thorough exploration of each of these areas. As each person is unique, each reader will approach the book in his or her own way and will need different ingredients to increase their sense of vitality, which Dr Rowe's VitalityMark assessment will help to identify.

It is an honour and delight to be a colleague and friend of Dr Rowe's. I know you will enjoy *The Vitality Mark*, as his book comes to help save the day, save your life and, most importantly, add life to your years as well as your days.

Beth Frates

MD FACLM DipABLM

Acknowledgements

As the saying goes, it takes a village to raise a child, and it certainly takes support to write a book. For me, much of this support was intangible and invisible, as I had told virtually no one that I was starting to write it. This gave me the freedom to simply write and keep going, without distraction or being asked, 'When will it be finished?' However, there are a number of people whose quiet encouragement was very much heard by me.

Ray Sinnott, my friend who 'minds' the beautiful Mount Congreve Gardens close to where I live, whose warm invitations deepened my interest in the natural world and mindful environments in general. Immersing myself regularly in the essence of this most generative of spaces boosted my creativity and further sparked my curiosity for vitality.

My late mum and dad, Brendan and Geraldine, who gave me the best of starts in life: a loving home and a great education. I miss them both dearly, and would love more than anything to show them this book. I know they are still 'there' watching over me, and in moments of stillness and silence, I clearly feel their presence.

Margaret, an elderly patient so full of spirit despite her depleted physical health. She had read my *Prescription for Happiness* book several years earlier, and her forensic enquiries as to when was I going to write 'the next one' sparked seeds of creativity in me. Thank you, Margaret, for your gentle encouragement.

To my many patients who have had the courage to take action and become more active participants in their own wellbeing. I'm grateful to all of you, as you fuel my purpose and inspire me to further leverage my messages of positive health.

Of course, I'm grateful to the gift of science and frontline workers everywhere who have done so much throughout the Covid-19 pandemic. Closer to home, my wonderful colleagues and practice team at the Rowe Creavin Medical Practice – your steadfast loyalty and dedication in the past few years has meant so much to me. A big thank you from me to all of you, particularly to my practice manager Julie.

Special thanks to the team at Gill Books for their professionalism, especially Rachel Thompson and Sarah Liddy, Teresa Daly and Claire O' Flynn.

Dr Beth Frates from Harvard Medical School, who wrote the foreword. Beth is a true pioneer of the lifestyle as medicine movement.

Dr Doireann O'Leary, who has generously supported and endorsed my messages of positivity.

The eclectic guests in my weekly podcast, *In the Doctor's Chair*, who have all encouraged and supported me and sparked meaningful reflections in their own way. I'm grateful to each and every one of you.

And finally, thanks to my wife, Edel, and children Malcolm, Tony and Lydia, who support me in everything.

Contents

Introduction

Imagine you feel energised and invigorated, when you might otherwise feel tired and depleted. Better able to withstand inflammation, illness and insidious disease. Your immune system reinforced, strengthening your natural defences against infection, while helping to buffer you from age-related degeneration. Your health span (the number of years you stay healthy) lengthened, and life added to your years. Your potential maximised.

As you become awake and alive to this possibility, your mind feels focused and clear. You become less reactive and more responsive as you develop crystal clarity in your decision-making. You wake in the morning with a sense of enthusiasm and optimism for a new day, fully present in the moment, finding joy in little things and a sense of flow in your lived experiences. You feel creative and more attuned to your senses and experiences, more connected to others. You care less about 'me' and more about 'we'. You choose to spend more time in health-enhancing environments. Your spiritual energy is high, with a deep sense of fulfilment and inner contentment. You know that what you do – and, more importantly, who you are – really does matter. You are fuelled by a strong sense of purpose and meaning.

For me, these are the elements that form the essence of living with vitality: an opportunity to think, feel and become the best possible version of you. Vitality, as a word, is defined as 'exuberant physical strength or mental vigour: a person of great vitality', or someone with 'capacity for survival or for the continuation of a meaningful or purposeful existence'. For me, vitality is a vibrant definition of wellbeing that incorporates the elements of emotion, physical health, mind, spirit and connection (in terms of relationships and environment) – all underpinned, of course, by a strong sense of purpose.

In Ancient Rome, Cicero wrote that philosophy teaches us to 'be doctors to ourselves'. To me, this represents an enlightened idea of self-care – not just in terms of the individual, but a much broader definition that includes how you connect with and care for others. This combination of service to others, aligned to self-care in terms of body, mind, emotion and spirit, is the best way I know to live with vitality.

Throughout my career to date as a medical doctor, what I've come to appreciate more than anything else about wellbeing can be summarised in the short phrase: **everything is connected**. I've learned how physical, mental, emotional and spiritual aspects of your wellbeing, along with your relationships, environment and sense of purpose, all impact your vitality in an interconnected, synergistic way. They all influence who you are, and who you become. Small, positive changes can have a multiplying effect on other areas, compounding over time to create a big difference. Because, yes, I've said it already, but it's worth repeating: everything is connected.

As I write this, the world is still undergoing a period of tremendous change and massive disruption. Covid-19 wreaked havoc on the health and everyday life of so many. The result: a surreal state of stress and fear, a sense of suspended animation, along with economic strife and concern over an uncertain future. I have tremendous respect for people who are able to smile through adversity and stay strong. I believe resilience starts the moment you acknowledge and accept the reality you find yourself in. Facing and embracing adversity leads to growth. Denying or suppressing it emotionally simply leads to more suffering. Acceptance becomes the new starting point from which to move forward, one step, one day at a time.

The paradox of Covid is that while everyday life changed for so many, the birds still sang sweetly, the sun still rose each morning, and nature remained as beautiful and effervescent as ever. Time alone to contemplate in nature has been a real gift for me – for my senses, spirit and sense of creative connection. It has opened up fresh understandings yet given rise to new questions.

As a family physician, this pandemic has impacted me in ways I never imagined, from conversations I've had with people, patients and myself to questioning and re-evaluating what matters most. A common theme in these conversations has been the importance of good 'health', including mind, body, emotion, spirit and connections. In short, life with vitality.

In a way, this book is my response to the pandemic. It is a paradigm shift from what you have lost to how you can grow as an active participant in your own wellbeing – rather than simply a passive consumer of healthcare. How to grow more in compassion, care and consideration to the needs of others as well as yourself. To understand that in any given moment you can choose how to respond. To choose to live with more vitality.

Your VitalityMark

The starting point, on this journey to living with more vitality, is to work out where you're beginning from. That's where my VitalityMark assessment comes in; it's a subjective, 'moment in time' online measurement of your current wellbeing. The questionnaire scores you separately in each of the five areas of your vitality – emotion, physical, spirit, mind and connection – in addition to giving you an overall vitality score: your own VitalityMark.

Your individual scores may signal which area is of most relevance to you right now. Perhaps it's your physical energy or attentive focus that needs the most attention; or maybe it's your sense of purpose. Whatever it is, the reality is that everyone has gaps. And VitalityMark is not about being perfect, but rather about progress. What gets measured gets improved, and the smallest of actions can speak so much more loudly than the smallest of intentions.

Perhaps most important of all, however, is the remembrance that everything is interconnected. This is one of the key principles of VitalityMark, and it's why improving any one element of your vitality may positively impact on other elements as well. VitalityMark supports you to become a more active participant in your own wellbeing and to express a more revitalised version of yourself in the world. The essence of VitalityMark as a wellbeing tool is that it allows you to identify and commit to adopting small, positive lifestyle habits that strengthen and support you in your self-care journey. It is *your* commitment to live with more vitality – to never stop starting.

Let's try to get a rough sense of your VitalityMark now, with a look at some sample questions that I use in my online assessment. Read through the following statements carefully and decide whether you agree or disagree with each one. Then try to think about whether your answers highlight any areas where you could be living with more vitality.

Emotion

- My life is filled with people and activities that interest and engage me
- I am optimistic about the future
- I never feel lonely or left out
- I am satisfied with my life overall

Physical

○   I get eight hours of sleep each night

○   I get at least 150 minutes of moderately intense exercise each week (able to talk but not sing) *or* at least 75 minutes of intense exercise each week (can neither talk nor sing)

○   I move regularly throughout the day

○   I eat a wide variety of plant-based foods (beans, peas, lentils, vegetables, fruit, whole grains, nuts and seeds)

Spirit

○   If I could live my life over, I would change very little

○   I spend some time daily in solitude or silence

○   My values are an important guide to my choices and decisions

○   I have a great sense of purpose and meaning in my life

Mind

○   I focus my attention on one thing at a time, not distracted by email, texts or social media

○   I keep a written journal for reflective purposes

○   Learning new things is important to me

○   I find it easy to switch off from work

Connection

○   I experience feelings of burnout

○   I spend time regularly in nature

○   I make enough time for my friends

○   I value the importance of self-care

This is only a short, unscored sample of my VitalityMark assessment, but these are questions that everybody can benefit from thinking about consciously. And, as I've said, the aim of the measurement is progress – so it may be helpful to return to this section once you've finished this book and see if your answers have changed at all.

To learn more about VitalityMark, including how to get a full, accurate measurement of your current VitalityMark and benefit from associated resources, log on to drmarkrowe.com.

AGEING WELL

While knowledge cares about answers, wisdom is more interested in asking the right questions. By combining objective data from science, aligned to subjective experience in my work as a medical doctor, I believe that asking the right questions has never been more important. Questions that include:

○   Why do people suffer from toxic stress and anxiety?

○   Why do many people neglect their own self-care needs?

○   Why do some people grow older without the decrepitude of ageing?

According to the World Health Organization, two-thirds or more of all diseases worldwide will soon be the result of lifestyle habits. Currently, the leading causes of death in the United States are all lifestyle-related: poor diet, lack of exercise, obesity, tobacco use and overconsumption of alcohol.

In recent decades, the lifestyle habits of the Western World have contributed to a tsunami of chronic health conditions, from diabetes and dementia to coronary heart disease and countless others. An epidemic of anxiety, addiction and mental health conditions has emerged, with more people than ever searching for purpose and meaning. Conventional healthcare has traditionally embraced 'a pill for every ill', and the mindset on ageing is equated with retirement and the associated inexorable decline into senility.

When patients attend me in my practice, the computerised record tells me their 'age' and date of birth. Of course, no one can change this number staring out from the computer; your date of birth or **chronological age** is fixed – for you, for me, for all of us! But what I call your **biological age** – the miles on your clock – that's a different story. Something that has intrigued me for many years is how older people with similar dates of birth can simply look and be so different in terms of their health. Could it simply be down to bad luck or genetics?

Well, an answer has been provided by a Danish twin study which found that only about 20 per cent of the difference in the health of identical twins was down to genetics. The remaining 80 per cent related to environmental and lifestyle differences[1].

In medical school, we learn that our DNA is set in stone. Untouchable, unchangeable. That our biological blueprint determines our destiny. While part of a person's genome clearly does remain fixed, perhaps up to 80 per cent of how your genes express themselves is regulated by something called your **epigenome**. The Greek word *epi* means 'upon', so epigenetics is essentially the study of what sits on top of genetics. The epigenome is the sheath of proteins and chemicals that cushions, protects and modifies each strand of your DNA. It can be switched on or off like a light switch, up and down like a thermostat. Furthermore, your epigenetics are influenced largely by your lifestyle. Therefore, assuming a fair wind and an element of good fortune (it always helps!), and within the confines of biological limits (which, for age, is thought to be about 100 for most people and up to 120 for outliers), then all things being equal, the healthiest lifestyle can be expected to maximise your life expectancy.

In other words, your genetic expression (excepting hereditary conditions) is to a large measure under your own control and responds to the lifestyle choices you make and the environments you experience each and every day of your life. Expressing your epigenetic potential in a health-enhancing way can help slow the ageing process, enhance your energy, normalise your metabolism and decrease your risk of developing many chronic diseases. Every day in my surgery, I see epigenetics in action when I meet people who look much older (or younger) than their age. In fact, many 'elderly' citizens over the age of 85 are much, much younger biologically (75, max). This is a big change from when I started in practice, when someone surviving to, never mind thriving at, age 85 was something of a rarity. The bottom line is that you have two ages, chronological and biological, and what I've learned from my experience to date is that your biological age is heavily influenced by your lifestyle.

The Dunedin Study, headed up by Duke University, tracked almost a thousand people from New Zealand born in 1972 and 1973 and calculated their biological age after their 38th birthday. While there is currently no definitive measure of biological age, the researchers used 18 separate biomarkers (including dental health, cholesterol levels, brain health, condition of blood vessels at the back of the eye) as well as other tests, including measures of balance and muscle strength. The researchers found that while most people aged by one biological year for each chronological year, some people aged much slower or faster than this. The biological age of the participants varied from 28 to 61! Some participants aged by as much as three years for each chronological year, and these people not only looked older but had evidence of brain ageing and generalised decline as well.

Blue zones are areas of the world where longevity is the rule rather than the exception; where people have a threefold increased chance of living to be 100. Not simply striving to or surviving, but actually thriving well beyond age 90 in every sense of what it means to be human. It turns out that inhabitants of these areas have a number of features in common. These include a largely plant-based or Mediterranean diet, regular movement and exercise, an ability to recharge from stress, in addition to connections with friends, community, having a strong sense of purpose, and a higher power. These areas include the Nicoya Peninsula in Costa Rica, the Barbagia region of Sardinia in Italy, Okinawa in Japan and the Greek island of Icaria.

While not many of us can choose to emigrate to these parts of the world, in reality, you don't have to. By integrating positive health principles with the promising science of lifestyle as medicine, aligned to my practical tips, you can gift yourself more vitality in your everyday experiences, and your longer-term wellbeing.

LIFESTYLE AS MEDICINE

The idea of lifestyle habits as effective medicine is very old. Just think of Hippocrates ('let food be your medicine and medicine your food'), or Cicero ('it is exercise alone that supports the spirits and keeps the mind in vigour') among many others espousing the many benefits. More recently, Thomas Edison wrote: 'The doctor of the future will give no medicine, but instead will interest his patients in the care of the human frame, in diet and in the cause and prevention of disease.' That future is now arriving, with the principles of lifestyle medicine gaining real traction around the world, underpinned by a growing body of scientific evidence. This is bringing to life the idea of taking care of your body as though you might really need it for one hundred years.

The European Prospective Investigation into Cancer and Nutrition (EPIC) study, involving almost 25,000 men and women, found that the presence of four healthy lifestyle factors – not smoking, normal weight, moderate exercise of at least 30 minutes per day, and a high intake of vegetables, fruit and whole grains with low meat intake – reduced the risk of chronic disease by 78 per cent. Another study by the Harvard

School of Public Health found that people who exercised an average of 30 minutes a day, never smoked, didn't drink alcohol to excess, weren't overweight and ate a healthy diet lived an additional 12 to 14 years on average![2]

The Harvard Study of Adult Development expands on these findings, listing six factors that are associated with healthy ageing – exercise, not smoking (or drinking alcohol to excess), healthy weight, healthy coping mechanisms with stress, stable mood and (in inner-city deprived areas) education which supports positive lifestyle change.

Mindset about ageing matters too, big time! Yale University research has found that simply having a positive view of ageing (seeing growing older as an opportunity to gain wisdom and fresh perspectives) as opposed to a negative view of ageing (sense of loss, disability) can support you to live at least seven years longer[3].

This concept of a healthy lifestyle as a helping hand for more vitality has captivated me for years. The environments you spend your time in can be either health-enhancing or health-depleting – not just the outer environments you work and live in, but the inner environments of thought and emotion. All underpinned by a strong sense of purpose: knowing that what you do and who you are really does matter.

As a doctor, I'm a scientist at heart, swayed by the evidence. For me, this has two separate interrelated elements. First, randomised controlled trials and other pieces of objective research, some of which I have mentioned. Second, I also value subjective experience in terms of what I see in my surgery each day, and how my suggestions and strategies to improve health can have an impact.

IN MY PRACTICE

Which brings me to John, the quintessential doctor-avoiding Irish male. I met him for the first time when he was 70 years old and was legally required to see his doctor to have his driver's licence renewed. While his wife had been regularly attending our practice for many years, this was our first time to meet up. It was John's first time with a doctor 'for as long as [he] could remember'. Even though he had access to free medical care by virtue of his medical card, that clearly hadn't been enough to entice him to avail of the occasional check-up.

With the formalities of the driver's licence dispensed with, I dug into his lifestyle. Very sedentary, no exercise worth talking about, little enough movement throughout his day. Poor eating habits with plenty of takeaways loaded with salt and fat, washed down with 'slabs of beer' at the weekends. Unsurprisingly, his blood pressure was up. He looked every day of his 70 years. Biologically, he was at least 77.

'At least you don't smoke,' I said, gently cajoling him into having some simple blood tests with a planned review scheduled for a week later. The results revealed what I suspected: a ticking time bomb. Blood pressure high. Raised total and LDL (bad) cholesterol, raised blood fat and low HDL (good) cholesterol. Raised blood sugar and ninety-day blood sugar test (HbAlc) putting him in the diabetes range.

Raised liver function tests suggesting fatty liver disease. Raised uric acid suggesting attacks of gout were on the way. Belly circumference of 44 inches, confirming the presence of metabolic syndrome, a condition that puts you at significantly increased risk of stroke, heart disease and diabetes. I didn't know where to start!

'To be honest John,' I said, 'you need treatment for your blood pressure, diabetes and cholesterol. We are talking about at least six tablets a day and that's just for starters. But there is an alternative. No guarantees, but if you can make major lifestyle changes, then you will be able to avoid at least some of the medication.'

To my genuine and great surprise, John said that's what he wanted to do. We had a conversation about what needed to happen next as part of a ninety-day simple action plan. Cut out the slabs of beer. Move as much as possible. Eat real food, lots of colour, mainly vegetables and fruit. Most importantly, stay on track. If you have the odd slip, don't worry, just get back on track again as soon as you can. Focus on progress, not perfection.

As planned, John had his bloods rechecked and came back for a review appointment, without needing to call him in. Six months after our initial meeting, his results were now astonishingly good. Diabetes reversed. Liver function normal. Blood fat and cholesterol back in normal range. Uric acid normal. On examination, his blood pressure was down. He had taken more than four inches off his belly circumference.

He said he felt great, with much more energy, and felt his mood had improved as well. Of note, his subjective wellbeing (a score between zero and ten in terms of his perceived mood) was seven out of ten. When I had met him first, he had said it was five (not depressed, but certainly flat). He said he was sleeping better, and he wasn't waking up feeling tired in the mornings any longer. Perhaps best of all, he looked terrific – much younger, with a real vibrancy about him.

What had John really done after my advice was dispensed? That's what interests me, because actions speak louder than words. John had walked the walk. He loaded up on fresh vegetables and only ate food from his own kitchen. He made regular pots of vegetable soup and stews with lots of chopped sweet potatoes, chickpeas and lentils to bulk them out. Committed to eating and drinking nothing after six o'clock in the evening, apart from some herbal tea. Made sure never to shop when hungry and stopped buying treats 'just in case we have visitors'. Ditched the slabs of beer. Started walking, firstly the 10 minutes or so to and from the local shop instead of driving, then built the walking habit until he was averaging about 12,000 steps a day. Perhaps best of all, he took my advice to buy an exercise bike. Piggybacking exercise with his favourite hobby of watching some TV at night, he quickly built up to more than an hour or more each day on the bike. He brought micro-moments of movement into his day. When sitting down watching TV, he committed to standing up and walking around during every commercial break.

I was delighted to celebrate John's achievements with him. Not so much the blood results per se, more that he had chosen to become an active participant in his own wellbeing, as opposed to being a passive consumer of healthcare. That commitment by John had made all the difference. Furthermore, he spoke about how he was now actively encouraging his wife to become healthier. This was the ripple effect of positive lifestyle changes in evidence before my own eyes.

John and I have joked since about how he has become my 'poster boy' for positive lifestyle change. I'm proud to know John and for his efforts to improve his own health. It's never easy to change the habits of a lifetime, but can be so worthwhile, especially when it comes to your greatest asset, your health.

IN WITH THE OLD

The conventional concept of health is defined through the lens of illness: if you're not sick or feeling unwell, then your health is fine. What I've learned is that health is so much more than just the absence of disease. Good health is a priceless gift, the greatest gift of all. More than 70 years ago, in 1948, the World Health Organization (WHO) defined health as not merely the absence of disease, but a state of complete physical, mental and relational wellbeing. Unfortunately, this statement has gathered dust for far too long. It's only recently that elements of the medical profession are 'waking up' to this WHO definition.

In life we are all formed by our own experiences. For me, the aftermath of the 2009 financial crash fundamentally changed how I viewed 'health'. With a deluge of people suffering from fear, financial pressure and toxic stress now attending me in my medical practice, it rapidly became apparent that people needed – more than pills – hope and what I call realistic optimism – understanding that things can improve through the power of your own efforts. Let me be clear: this was not an attempt to denigrate or pooh-pooh the potential benefits of medication for many health conditions (including depression and anxiety). Far from it. Rather it was a growing awareness that, on its own, medication was not enough. While talk therapy can be invaluable, at that time it was only available if you could pay. This was the eureka moment that prompted me to research additional ways to support my many patients who were struggling or suffering. It led to my interest in learning more about the potential benefits of positive psychology interventions and how prescribing positive lifestyle changes as 'medicine' can make such a difference in the health, wellbeing and everyday lived experience for many.

For me to effectively embrace this truth, I needed to look backwards to look forwards. In 2017, Gensler (a global architecture, design and planning firm) hosted me at their headquarters in Washington, DC for several days to address their clients and staff about wellbeing. While there, I was introduced through a fascinating conversation with someone to the *Tao Te Ching*, a classic Chinese text written by Lao Tzu. I had heard of Lao Tzu (who famously wrote that 'the journey of a thousand miles begins with a single step'), but the teachings of the *Tao Te Ching* were completely new territory for me. When I got back home to Ireland, I immediately ordered a copy of the text to learn more.

Dating back to pre-Confucian times (about 400 BC), the essence of the *Tao* essentially concerns a way of being in the world where 'being', rather than knowing or having, is the highest order there is. My key takeaways were that it espouses inner integrity, a sense of balance, proportion and a way of living that is in harmony with nature and the world you live in. By emphasising the importance of simplicity, universal compassion and humility, it also highlights that emotional energy connects in turn to physical, spiritual and mental energy. In other words, it shows how interconnected the various elements of your wellbeing really are.

Bearing this ancient philosophy in mind, I then began looking forward again, to embrace the environment of the epigenome, habits that help health span and support living with more vitality. It may have taken many years of practising the 'old way' for me to wake up to this new reality, but as they say, better late than never. What's even better is that once you see things differently, then there's no going back to the old way.

Personal reflections, as well as professional observation of and interaction with my patients over many years, has enabled me to open my eyes to this concept of vitality. That's what this book is about: an opportunity for me to share what I've learned so far in giving you knowledge, skills and ideas to reset your course towards habits that are more health-enhancing and revitalising. In turn, you may become an even more positive influence on those people around you, as well as have fun along the way.

Using this book

Perhaps the most important (even the only) question for you to answer right now is: why read this book? Whether you are struggling with your wellbeing, or simply looking to further enhance your vitality, then this book is for you.

The book is broken into sections that can be read either sequentially or on a stand-alone basis. My promise is that you will learn some science-based strategies and suggestions to live with more vitality. This book is about those small changes that stick, from the inside out. Not massive changes, but simply appreciating the potential that comes from thinking small, and that small positive changes over time can make a real difference.

The book is broken into four parts: the heart, body, soul and mind of vitality. As I've already said, my belief is that all areas of our health are intrinsically connected, and each part of the book will focus on strategies and techniques that can lead to improvements in each part of your life. I have also included case studies to illustrate how these concepts have worked in my practice – real-life examples of patients who derived benefit from lifestyle changes.

There are also sections throughout the book where I ask you to engage in personal reflection. Keeping a written journal can be invaluable to become really clear about your goals and your written plan for achieving them. It teaches you objective perspective, enabling you to see things more clearly and to evaluate your progress. A good intention is far more likely to result in action with advance planning and proper preparation. For example, it can be helpful to reflect on what worked for you before and why. What could go better next time and how? What are the situations, people and places that can provide support (or indeed hinder) your proposed change?

Reviewing each week in this way allows your unfolding experiences to become the best curriculum to learn from. Leveraging your own previous successes and 'failures', planning for success while anticipating roadblocks and challenges can support you in making lasting change. This is perhaps the best way to make sustainable progress towards any worthwhile life change. Fail to prepare, prepare to fail!

Living your life through the lens of 'vitality' has many benefits. You will think, feel and become closer to your creative best, expressing a better version of yourself in the world.

IN MY PRACTICE

I saw this clearly with a recent patient of mine, Richard, who attended me for a series of lifestyle consultations. He had taken my wellbeing assessment tool, and his overall score was 60 per cent – reasonably good, with plenty of room for improvement. VitalityMark had provided him with a written pdf and targeted video resources, based on how he had answered. One recommendation was for him to keep a written journal.

Richard hadn't written anything down regularly since homework assignments at school, decades earlier. Yet he was now curious about the potential benefits of keeping a written journal, termed 'thinking on paper' and so loved by philosophers of old, especially given that it didn't require much time, just a few minutes each day. Richard began by writing down his main health goals for the week in terms of his exercise and eating habits and then simply tracked each day what actually happened.

What's interesting is that the executive and writing parts of the brain are located close together, which is why written goals can be so affirming. Actions speak louder than words, of course, written or otherwise. Reviewing his progress each week was key to enabling Richard to become crystal clear about how he was matching up. Learning what had gone well and why, as well as those days when he had fallen short, allowed his own experiences to become a template for potential improvement. By getting to know himself better, he became more aware of his intention gaps, as well as the people, places, environments and situations that supported his health goals. This habit of self-reflection supported Richard to make lasting improvements over time. In his own words, he became 'more aware of what I was really doing each day, and by holding myself accountable, naturally became more active and a healthier eater over time. For such a simple idea, the journal can have a big impact. It did for me anyway and I'd highly recommend anyone to give it a try and see if it works for them.'

THE HAND OF VITALITY

I developed this Hand of Vitality model as a practical means of, firstly, better understanding just how interconnected the various elements of your vitality are. Secondly, it can also help you to appreciate that living with more vitality is about simplicity, how small changes can lead to big improvements over time. Small positive changes in one element of your vitality provide a multiplicity of benefits in other elements. Take a look at your own hand: try and picture where each element fits in as you read through the descriptions below, and as you read through this book. The Hand of Vitality provides an opportunity to know yourself well enough to discover those elements of the model that can work best for you.

○ **Little Finger: The Heart of Vitality**
The little finger represents emotional essence, the heart of vitality. Its three segments are the art of gratitude, the act of kindfulness and flourishing emotional energy – an antidote to negativity.

○ **Ring Finger: The Body of Vitality**
The ring finger represents physical energy, or the body of vitality. Its three segments are restorative sleep, exercise and mindful eating.

○ **Middle Finger: The Soul of Vitality**
The middle finger represents spiritual essence, the soul of vitality. Its three segments are purpose, meditation and nature.

THE HAND OF VITALITY

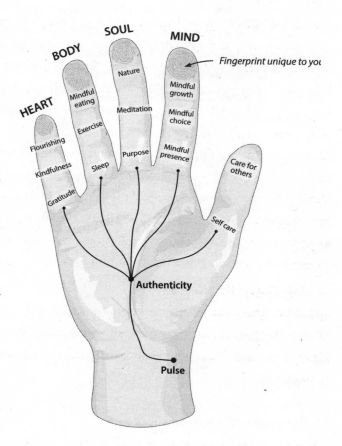

○ Index Finger: The Mind of Vitality

The index finger represents mental energy, the mind of vitality. Its three segments are mindful presence, mindful choice and mindful growth.

○ **Thumb: Self-care**

The thumb is a reminder of the fundamental importance of self-care. Its two segments are self-care and care for others. As you extend your hand to others, the base of your thumb points towards *you*, highlighting the importance of self-care; taking good care of yourself as a starting point to sustainably support others in your life.

○ **Centre of Your Hand**

Purpose, located at the base of your middle finger, connects to the centre of your hand as a reminder of the importance of authenticity. Authentic connection engages you with the essence of who you are – raw, unscripted and real.

○ **Fingerprint**

Your Hand of Vitality has a unique fingerprint – *yours*! A reminder that you are a unique individual, with the likelihood of two people sharing identical fingerprints by chance estimated to be less than one in 64 billion. Do you appreciate just how unique and special you are?

○ **The Area Around Your Hand**

The area around your hand represents the environments you spend your time in. These environments can either be health-enhancing or health-depleting. They can influence your emotions, body, spirit, mind and indeed your self-care as well as your connection with others.

Your second hand represents attitudinal and emotional

contagion. The mirror neurons in your brain lead to you being influenced by those people you spend most time with, in person or online. Emotional contagion means that emotion can spread outwards to three degrees of separation.

○ Pulse

The pulse represents the vibrancy and positive energy that you can bring to the world through the interconnection of the various elements of your vitality. A reminder to become more of an active participant in your own wellbeing, as opposed to simply a passive consumer of healthcare.

○ Movement

Your hand can open and close, flex and extend, pronate and supinate (these latter two being medical terms that describe whether your hand is in an up – supinated – or down – pronated – position). This reflects the fact that your vitality is neither constant nor static, but remains open to change and improvement.

CLOSING THE INTENTION GAP

Anne Frank wrote that our lives are fashioned by our choices; first we make our choices, and then they make us. Over time, the self-care habits you cultivate and everyday choices you make all add up to influence the person you become. For better *and* (unfortunately) for worse. Perhaps this is why making lasting change in your life can be so challenging, as you tend to stay thinking, feeling and doing what you have always thought, felt and done. The opportunity, I believe, is in joining the dots, connecting how you think and feel with what you do and how you behave. If you want to live with more vitality, chances are you are going to have to bridge the gap between who you are right now and a more revitalised version of you – your **intention gap**.

One of greatest lessons I've learned as a doctor is that knowledge does not equate to action – there is always a potential intention gap between what you could do and what you actually do. You may fool yourself into thinking that you will start to build healthier habits at some unspecified future date. That there's no rush in starting, since you've got all the time in the world. This '*mañana* mindset' can create significant inertia to change. While you may well know that you *could* change, and perhaps that you *should* change, you simply don't. Furthermore, you may well actively resist change (even if this is at a subconscious level) due to your biological programming.

Homeostasis is this inbuilt tendency of your brain, body and behaviour to resist change. It is an important survival mechanism: the ongoing tweaking and recalibration of billions of interconnected neurons and associated neurochemicals that continually interact to maintain an inner state of equilibrium. From blood sugar levels to body temperature and thousands of other processes, the maintenance of inner balance or homeostasis is a key survival tool.

The problem is that homeostasis doesn't distinguish between good and bad change. It resists them all! Which is why making positive lifestyle changes can be so challenging. As a result of homeostasis, people can generate a lot of toxic stress, triggering feelings of fear and anxiety by resisting change. Homeostasis means you are hardwired to instinctively resist change by keeping you within your comfort zone, believing you are safe and secure in doing what you've always done, not needing to take on new challenges. Now, comfort zones may be nice places, but nothing of consequence ever grows there.

One of the great things about change, of course, is that life is continually changing. Every single day, millions of cells in your body change. Your red blood cells change every four months, skin cells change every few days. Even 10 per cent of the cells in your bones change each year.

But still, bridging the intention gap through change isn't easy. As the saying goes, the road to hell is paved with good intentions. As a doctor, I meet so many people who know what to do in terms of improving their health and vitality, and may intend to do something about it, but they still don't close the gap to make positive behavioural change. This gap is real for everyone and doesn't mean you are weak, lazy or lacking in character – simply that you are human, with all that entails.

What's your barrier to taking the first step and simply starting? Perhaps you believe this change is not that important – nice to do maybe, but not needed right now. Perhaps you feel too busy, too tired or stressed. Perhaps you procrastinate until some more opportune or 'perfect time' in the future. Perhaps you don't appreciate just how difficult changing your existing patterns of behaviour can be.

Intention to change on its own is not nearly enough to result in the desired change. In fact, research suggests it only accounts for about 25 per cent of the variation in why some people do or don't move and eat healthily. Common sense is rarely common action! In terms of closing your intention gap, here are some questions to reflect on before we move on to strategies to support your success.

Journal

Consider an aspect of your vitality that you'd like to change for the better.

O   Why do you want to bring this positive change into your life?

O   How important is this change to you?

O   How confident are you of success?

O   List three compelling reasons to take action.

O   What value will this new vitality habit bring to your life?

O   What worked for you before and why?

O   What could go better this time and how?

O   What excuses will you no longer accept?

O   How can you redesign your environments at home or at work to support this new commitment?

O   Who can support, strengthen and encourage you (in person and/or virtually)? In turn, who can you support and mentor along the way?

O   How are you going to measure and celebrate success?

O   What's the smallest step you can take to move in the direction you want to go in?

There's an African saying that resonates with me in terms of the intention gap: 'If there's no enemy within, then the enemy outside can do you no harm; while you can outrun what's beside you, you can't outrun what's inside of you.'

Why do you want to bring this positive change into your life? As they say, if you know your why, the how gets easier. Answering these questions can create a tipping point towards positive change.

How important is this change to you and how confident are you that you can achieve it? Research from motivational interviewing suggests that scoring yourself at least seven out of ten for each of these two questions significantly increases the chances of successful change[4]. If it's not important to you, why would you bother? If you score less than seven on this question of 'importance', then learning more about the potential benefits of the desired change can make all the difference. This is why I have written this book: to shine a light on lifestyle strategies that can support you to live with more vitality. If your 'confidence' score for making a change is less than seven, then having a detailed plan can be invaluable to support your success.

YOUR PERSONAL PRESCRIPTION

There's an African proverb that resonates with me: 'If you are running away from something, it means that something is chasing you.' Fear is generally a poor motivator of long-term positive change, particularly when it comes to health habits and lifestyle choices. It's one of the reasons why traditional medical advice can fall on deaf ears. Fear of getting diabetes or heart disease at some point in the future is unlikely to get you off the couch this evening. Similarly, stopping smoking now to prevent lung cancer in the future may be pretty self-evident, but unlikely to be enough to encourage most smokers to stop. Even thinking about lung cancer may increase feelings of fear, anxiety and toxic stress, leading to yet another cigarette. If someone has a heart attack, they are likely to do whatever their doctor tells them for about a month. After that time interval, however, the fear wears off as you adapt to the 'new normal' and may well revert to type in terms of your pre-existing lifestyle habits.

Before we get down to work, here are a few personal prescriptions as we begin this journey together. Considering these factors will increase your chances of long-term success in living a life of vitality.

Grow your grit: In Aesop's fable, the hare looks disparagingly at the pace of the plodding tortoise, who challenges the hare to a race as a result. At the start, the hare sprints away into the distance, so far ahead of the slow tortoise that it stops for a nap midway. Awakening many hours later, it finds the tortoise is close to the finish line, and, despite its best efforts, is unable to catch up.

What about you? Are you more a tortoise or a hare? Do you live your life like a marathon or a series of short sprints? Do you stay the course you have committed to? Do you keep going even when passed out by people that are younger, stronger, faster? In a world of so much choice and distraction, it's so easy to live like the hare. The hare lives by the myth of natural talent; the fixed mindset which doesn't value effort. The tortoise epitomises grit and the growth mindset, emphasising 'one small step at a time', in addition to sustained effort over time.

In 1940, *TIME* magazine profiled the bravado and tenacity of Finnish spirit, in the face of relentless oppression during World War II[5]. In Finland, they name this trait *sisu* (pronounced see-sue). It is their sense of courage, hardiness and stoic determination – an inner strength, fortitude and perseverance. More than 80 per cent of Finns have a growth mindset about the development of *sisu*. It becomes a self-reinforcing behaviour, symbolising an unquenchable spirit, that comes from vulnerability in the face of adversity. As the essence of grit, *sisu* can be a tremendous strength, but like everything, it's about the sweet spot of balance. Too much *sisu* can trigger exhaustion or burnout, so it must be balanced with self-compassion, empathy and acceptance.

Grit is defined by psychologist Angela Duckworth in her bestselling book of the same name as a combination of passion and sustained persistence for a singularly important goal, without regard to recognition or reward. The essence of grit is to fall seven times and get up eight, to keep putting one foot in front of the other. To have purposeful goals, passionate interest and to practise, practise, practise. To be uncomfortable being comfortable, unsatisfied being satisfied. Grit boosts perseverance, self-regulation and likelihood of success (perhaps twice as likely a predictor of success than

IQ). Grit supports a healthier emotional life and more vitality.

Be patient and persistent: Research from University College London shows it takes 66 days on average to build a new habit, at which point it becomes easier to keep going with your new habit than to let go of it[6]. That's 66 days of committing to exercise even when you feel too tired, or believe you're too busy, or it's wet and windy outside. Furthermore, many attempts at change tend to fail after an initial 'honeymoon period' of a week or two when you revert to type, which is why having a strategy to deal with setbacks is so important. How will you deal with setbacks? You are not a machine or a mere key performance indicator of economic endeavour. You are a human being, with all your fascinations and foibles, flawed, but in many ways perfect in your imperfections. Speed bumps are inevitable along the way. Anticipate setbacks (people, places and situations) where your new commitment may be derailed. Having a detailed plan to navigate these can be invaluable to keep you on track.

Seek support: Who can support you in making this positive change? Joining a group with shared interests and common goals can be invaluable, with an element of group accountability as well. The people you spend time with can have a big influence on your lifestyle choices and health habits. In fact, the mirror neurons in the brain which, thousands of years ago, helped to keep you safe in a world full of danger and threats, encourage you to adopt the habits, attitudes and mannerisms of the people you spend most time with – right throughout your life, not just when you are a teenager. So if you spend time with people who eat healthily and exercise regularly, chances are you're going to eat healthily and exercise regularly as well. On the other hand, if you spend a lot of time with people with less-than-healthy lifestyle habits, chances are you're going to adopt some of those unhealthy habits as well. Furthermore, emotion is highly contagious and your emotional state has a significant impact on your everyday choices. This is why it is helpful to have people around you who will encourage and support you.

Consider willpower: Traditionally, willpower has been considered a badge of honour worn by people who successfully resisted temptation and were successful in making lifestyle changes. Those who didn't or couldn't say no simply had weaker willpower or were seen as being lazier, less committed or lacking in some way. But fascinating research by eminent psychologist Roy Baumeister in the late 1990s led to a paradigm shift in the understanding of willpower. In what is known as the 'Chocolate and Radish Experiment', three separate groups were asked to fill in a questionnaire before being taken to a separate room to solve a maths puzzle. Two of the groups had a bowl of (delicious-smelling) chocolate chip cookies and a bowl of radishes in front of them while they filled in the questionnaire. The first group was told they could eat the radishes but not the cookies as they were being kept for another experiment. The second group was told they could eat either the cookies or radishes, while the third group had no snacks available to them. After 15 minutes, each group was taken to a separate room to attempt the puzzle (unknown to the participants, this was an impossible puzzle to solve, and the psychologists wanted to see how long each group persisted). The results found that the two groups who had been offered either no snacks at all or the cookies and radishes persisted twice as long on the puzzle as the group that was denied the cookies (19 versus 8 minutes). This group's ability to persist with the puzzle was weakened because their willpower had been depleted in resisting the delicious-smelling chocolate chip cookies. This research highlights that willpower is a highly depletable resource with perhaps as little as 15 minutes of it available at any one time. Just consider the many aspects of daily decisions that require your willpower – emails, food choices, housework – and you will begin to see how valuable it is to plan in advance, to streamline and simplify your choices to better protect and manage your available willpower.

Celebrate success: Finally, it's important to celebrate the successes along the way. Reward yourself often as a reminder of your new commitment to your vitality. Making sustainable change isn't easy, and consumes a lot of mental energy. There's a saying: people tend to overestimate what they can achieve in one year and underestimate what they can achieve in five years. The key to long-term progress is consistency.

So, now that we've looked at the foundations we'll be looking to build – let's begin!

The Heart of Vitality

The heart of vitality is grateful, optimistic, open and kind – rich in empathy and compassion. At its essence, the heart of vitality has a reservoir of emotional positivity to make the most of good times and the resilience to respond to tough times, with a tipping point for flourishing in your personal life and interpersonal relationships.

It enables you to embrace more positive emotion and find flow experiences with a sense of enthusiasm, feeling more creative, curious and connected to others. You let go of the past and stories that no longer serve you, while appreciating the people and the things that are good right now and anticipating a more positive future.

The art of gratitude

'Gratitude turns what we have into enough.'

AESOP

The word 'gratitude' is derived from Latin *gratis*, meaning gratefulness or thankfulness. Take a moment to think about something you feel grateful for right now. Not just the last time you simply said please or thank you. While manners matter, they refer more to 'gratitude lite' than the real thing. True gratitude is a thank you with meaning, a thoughtful and intentional way of showing up in the world through the lens of appreciation. Taking notice of those little things that, at the end of the day, aren't so little.

Feeling grateful can flutter and flow with your mind, whereas being grateful is a conscious choice. As highlighted by philosophers from Seneca to Cicero, gratitude is an action, a practice of noticing and valuing, acknowledging and appreciating the actions of others. A commitment to channelling your energy into what's present and working rather than what's absent and ineffective. The art of true gratitude is to want what you have right now in your life, and not to simply have what you want. When you want what you already have, you appreciate the value of what you have as opposed to depreciating the value. As you appreciate the value of something, you are simply far less likely to take it for granted.

The practice of gratitude creates an upward spiral of wellbeing, whereby the more good things you see, the more good things you *will* see. Think of your mind as a garden, containing beautiful plants and weeds. Growing gratitude is an ongoing practice that's nurtured, cultivated and developed like a beautiful plant, enabling you to appreciate what you have right now – before time forces you to appreciate what you once had.

A group of Tibetan monks, who arrived in the USA to help determine whether meditative practice had influenced brain structure[7], expressed extreme surprise when the researchers wanted to scan their heads. Their belief was that the area around their hearts was far more relevant!

Gratitude has been described as the heart's way of remembering, the yin and yang between giving and receiving. It is heartfelt and comes from the heart. With gratitude you move from your head to your heart along the vagus nerve and in so doing move away from stress, engaging instead with the pause and plan relaxation response. Gratitude is powerful medicine to elevate your mood and fill you with joy, a natural antidote to feelings of toxic stress and 'chronic not-enoughness'. Gratitude brings perspective to the past, peace to the present and a sense of hope for the future.

If only it were that easy! In everyday life, there are many reasons why building the habit of gratitude sounds so easy yet can be so difficult. Gratitude takes effort. Many people become effortlessly self-absorbed in their own world, living with the illusion of self-sufficiency and self-serving bias. Of course, there are many reasons for this. People may simply be busy and time-pressed. Sometimes people become distracted, while some simply forget to be grateful.

Of course, as a creature of habit, you tend to think, feel and do what you've always thought, felt and done. It's so easy to forget about the many freedoms or material advantages that many people enjoy nowadays. The hardwired 'lizard brain', with its fear, survival and negativity bias, can detract from your potential to feel grateful. Especially if you, like many, are suffering from toxic stress. The human brain has an inbuilt tendency to take things for granted.

Gratitude Deficiency Syndrome is a term I use to describe the epidemic of expectancy that leads to negative comparison and envy. With the mindset of gratitude deficiency and entitlement, grievances will always outnumber gifts. Social media can foster feelings of inadequacy for failing to match up to so-called 'perfection'.

From simply taking things for granted to an excessive sense of self-importance, gratitude deficiency and its resultant emotional poverty are prevalent nowadays. A winner-takes-all mentality and material comparison underpins the celebrity culture of constant comment and comparison, while every mega dealmaker in the business world is cheered and copied. This can feed feelings of inadequacy and insecurity, particularly in those with low self-esteem.

Furthermore, the materialism of modern life results in many people taking these things for granted. Believing that the universe owes them a living can lead to feelings of expectancy and entitlement. This mindset can deplete you even further, even making you emotionally and spiritually bankrupt.

Epicurus once wisely wrote that people should remember that what they now have was once among the things they only hoped for. Entitlement and self-absorption can become major barriers, with the proverbial chip on the shoulder counteracting any tendency to gratitude.

Gratitude deficiency fosters the illusion of self-sufficiency, seeing success solely as a result of a person's own skills and hard work, unwilling to acknowledge the efforts of others or admit co-dependency. Compare this to the approach taken to life's setbacks, which are so often conveniently blamed on others.

Gratitude deficiency is a brain driven by greed and fear. Greed says 'give me more', fuelled by expectancy, entitlement and envy, while fear of not having enough or of not being enough is something I term 'chronic not-enoughness', that endless race of unfavourable comparison.

Entitlement says, 'I deserve this and I'm owed this. Life owes me.' Entitlement can lead to perceptions of unfairness, focusing on what one hasn't got, leading to resentment and envy of others when life fails to deliver for you. Bitterness, disillusionment, annoyance and anger, weighed down by feelings of needless negativity, can poison your world of thought, emotion and experience like a record constantly playing.

Eliminating entitlement by embracing gratitude can be emotionally, spiritually and psychologically liberating. Gratitude can become a powerful antidote to these thinking patterns. Grateful people are less materialistic. In fact, you can't be grateful and excessively materialistic at the same time, because a state of gratitude naturally lowers any tendency to materialistic thoughts.

Grateful people have less ego. They show more interest in others; and being better able to appreciate the achievements of others naturally makes people more likeable.

The brain likes novelty, newness and never stops adapting to our situation or circumstances. **Adaptation** is a remarkably resilient ability to rebound from setbacks and adversity, personal or professional. However, hedonic adaptation means you adapt and get used to the good things in life too. The result is that material benefits tend to have a short-lived impact as they become perceived as the new norm by your brain with something extra needed to provide the same level of satisfaction as before.

While gratitude can provide an antidote to help counteract this tendency to hedonic adaptation, what's interesting is how people adapt far more easily and quickly to material purchases than to experiences.

Because you are the sum of your total range of experiences, investing in experiences enhances who you are and tends to endure over time, unlike material purchases. Furthermore, experiences enable you to connect with others, leading to shared memories, strengthened relationships and longer-lasting satisfaction.

One of the great **myths about gratitude** is that it results in self-satisfied smugness, mediocrity and lack of grit and resolve. This is simply not true. Gratitude gives you more energy and vitality, fuelling purpose and persistence. An interesting study that grabbed my attention asked participants to set six personal goals to work on over a ten-week period[8]. Those also assigned a written gratitude journal (in which they were to write down five things they were grateful for, once a week) were found to exert more effort towards their goals, make 20 per cent more progress and to continue to work hard towards their goals afterwards. In other words, they didn't become complacent and self-satisfied in terms of impeding further progress. So gratitude is like a glue to support goal progress and build motivation. Gratitude supports efforts at self-improvement; when you feel encouraged and supported, you want to prove yourself worthy of those relationships.

Furthermore, gratitude is *not* about:

o   Ignoring your own hard work and efforts.

o   Having happy or positive thoughts always.

o   Ignoring the negative.

o   Indebtedness – 'You were good to me so now I owe you.'

BENEFITS OF GRATITUDE

Gratitude supports you to reframe and see the bigger picture in terms of recognising your own efforts **and** those people who have helped and supported you. From a medical perspective, expressing gratitude is so good for you that I consider it to be powerful medicine for your mind, body and soul. Putting on my medical hat for a moment, one of the great benefits of a regular gratitude habit is the ability to move away from impulsive reactivity and towards a more resilient response; to become less reactive and far more responsive to toxic stress.

An attitude of gratitude is a powerful antidote to needless negativity. Just as it is not possible to feel optimistic and pessimistic at the same time, it's not possible to feel negative, resentful and grateful at the same time. When you are feeling negative and stressed, the best treatment is a liberal dose of gratitude dispensed regularly.

Think about it like building an **emotional bank account**. As a positive emotion, gratitude feels good and increases subjective wellbeing. I consider gratitude to be a form of emotional dynamite, explosive in terms of how it transforms your thinking and expands your inner happiness. With gratitude, you experience more frequent positive emotions such as joy, optimism, enthusiasm and love, while dissolving anxiety and toxic negative stress. A gratitude practice may trigger negative emotion, especially early on when you may feel guilty, awkward or indebted, resulting in a paradox of temporary unhappiness. This is usually adaptive, however. As they say, 'short-term pain for longer-term gain'.

A gratitude practice can also be a significant happiness-boosting habit. Research has found that writing in a **gratitude journal** once a week for 10 consecutive weeks led to participants becoming up to 25 per cent happier[9]. A gratitude journal is a powerful way to boost your inner happiness and vitality. But it's a practice and personality trait which takes time to build, generally taking several months to become hardwired as a habit. While each journal entry on its own generates only very small amounts of positivity, it is enough to bring on a grateful mood. This allows you to recognise even more things to be grateful for and enhance recall of pleasant experiences, which in turn creates a positive feedback loop.

Gratitude can result in a more sustainable form of inner happiness as it results from a mindset shift away from the hardwired negative brain of instant gratification, towards heart-based real abundance. Through gratitude, you become much better able to savour good things and experiences. As a keystone habit for emotional vitality and emotional resilience, it can increase your capacity for joy and creativity and build a rich sense of contentment.

One of the things I have noticed as a doctor is that when asked, many people tell me that while they do feel grateful, they don't actually express it. Which is a pity; it's a bit like buying someone a gift and not giving it to them. While feeling grateful is certainly a good thing, to really experience the benefits it must be expressed. Writing it down crystallises your gratitude on paper so that it expands and enhances your awareness of the many good things in your life. It gives you context, a sense of meaning and makes it real.

Journal

What Went Well is a gratitude boosting exercise to remind your-self to write down three things each night you felt grateful for that day. Spend five to ten minutes reflecting on three things that went well – large or small – today, *and* why you think they happened.

By focusing on selecting positive things that are good in your life and happened today, you undertake a sort of filtering process whereby you filter out the more irrelevant and negative aspects. This retrains your brain to reinforce and better appreciate positive events in the future, which over time can lead to a real shift in your perspective and personal reality.

The key idea is that life, to a large degree, becomes how you choose to see it. This response – ability is your 'ability to respond' through the lens of gratitude and appreciation rather than absence and scarcity. Doing this simple What Went Well exercise every day for a week can increase happiness levels for up to six months subsequently.

Grateful relationships: Another benefit of gratitude is that the more grateful you are, the more likely you are to help others and to be seen by other people in your social network as being more helpful, as you become more socially engaged and motivated to help those around you.

There may be several reasons for this. Firstly, gratitude boosts inner happiness and vitality, both of which are associated with helping others. Secondly, gratitude opens up your heart to more kindness and compassion and boosts overall life satisfaction. It attunes your perceptiveness of kindness, which you will naturally then want to reciprocate. Thirdly, the grateful brain places more value on benefits to others, in terms of being kinder and paying it forward. As gratitude and kindness are interlinked, gratitude promotes generous giving. Gratitude helps you to see clearly how others have supported you, which encourages you to engage in positive actions to help others. It also encourages you to self-improve so as to be able to pay back those that have helped you.

There's a Russian proverb that says that 'Gratitude waters old friendships and makes new ones sprout'. Gratitude builds connection, feelings of being uplifted and optimism about humanity in general. Grateful people tend to be more friendly which encourages others to be more friendly too, building an upward spiral of social capital and strengthening your network of friends.

Gratitude is a rich relationship booster, a rechargeable magnetic force that produces greater connection with others. It awakens you to your interdependent nature: life is less about 'me' or 'you' and more about 'us' together. As such, it helps to combat feelings of loneliness and isolation.

THE SCIENCE OF GRATITUDE

Gratitude reorientates and rewires your brain towards what's positive and what's social. It changes the lens through which you see the world and combats the overdrive of both the 'hardwired negative brain' and hedonic adaptation. The health benefits of gratitude may be at least partly explained by plugging into those brain networks associated with stress relief and social connection.

According to UCLA's Mindful Awareness Research Center, expressing gratitude regularly can change the molecular structure of the brain, increasing grey matter volume in some areas (right inferior temporal gyrus). Gratitude can increase activity in the ventromedial prefrontal cortex, a key brain area for reward processing.

The USC Shoah Foundation has an archive of visual history that holds countless stories of selflessness and generosity amid the horrors of the Nazi death camps. In a study that looked at how feelings of gratitude correlate with brain activity, participants watched videos of hardship and imagined that they themselves had been there[10]. Next, gratitude was induced as they were shown a gift-giving scenario, for example, being given a warm coat to wear while in a death march in the height of winter or receiving some bread to eat while starving. Brain scans recorded any brain changes as the participants reflected deeply on their gratitude to be the beneficiary of such an act of kindness. Finally, they scored their perceived gratitude from one to four, with four being an overwhelming feeling of gratitude for the experience. FMRI (functional magnetic resonance imaging) brain scans were used to detect any change in brain activity throughout the experiment. The researchers found that specific brain areas are activated when gratitude is expressed, including areas that deal with regulation of emotion, empathy, social connection, fairness, perspective and stress relief.

As a personality trait, gratitude has been found to have a very strong association with life satisfaction and positive mental health[11]. Gratitude is strongly correlated with higher levels of optimism, as it trains the brain to see the future in a more optimistic light. It is a cornerstone of an attitude of positivity and possibility, supporting growth, grit and perseverance.

Gratitude broadens your perspective as you spend less and less mental energy distracted by worry, willpower control and needless negativity. This can free up some reserves in your subconscious mind to slow down and focus more of your attentive awareness on your work and whatever projects are right in front of you.

Just as your DNA is not set in stone, neither are your memories. Psychologist Danny Kahneman is perhaps best known for his fascinating research into cognitive biases, which has shown just how malleable your memories really are. It has also been suggested that expressing gratitude in the present moment can make you more likely to remember positive memories.

With a mindset of gratitude, you can learn to reframe setbacks and stressful life experiences in a more positive light, through the lens of growth, meaning and connection. This boosts resilience and more effective coping from stressors (minor and major).

Something worth considering is whether gratitude leads to good **physical health** or whether having good health leads to gratitude. Or perhaps there is some other variable influencing both gratitude and health? For example, gratitude may foster healthier lifestyle habits, more compliance with medical advice, and overall better levels of self-care. We know that gratitude is good for sleep (which in itself has health-boosting properties). In addition, gratitude is a great antidote to toxic stress, boosting positive emotions and happiness as well as strengthening relationships. All of these factors, alone or in combination, may help explain why gratitude can lead to better physical health.

People who have a gratitude practice report feeling healthier, with fewer aches and pains and increased subjective wellbeing. Appreciating your health encourages you to take active steps to stay healthy, including a regular check-up. This makes it easier to stick to a new exercise programme or other health-boosting habit.

The GRACE study – Gratitude Research in Acute Coronary Events – has found that grateful and optimistic people showed evidence of improved blood vessel function two weeks after suffering a heart attack. While no right-minded medic would suggest that gratitude alone can protect you from serious illness, it certainly does move you away from feelings of toxic stress towards relaxation and the parasympathetic nervous system which can help reduce your blood pressure and support your immune system.

Furthermore, this reduces the time taken to fall asleep, while improving sleep quality and duration. As I like to say, if you're having difficulty falling asleep, don't count sheep. Count your blessings instead! Research connects heartfelt appreciation with increased levels of salivary IgA[12] – the body's first line of defence against attack from invading microorganisms such as bacteria and viruses. Lower levels of cortisol can enhance healing and enable quicker recovery from illness. Gratitude may lead to the release of more endorphins, natural opioid painkillers that reduce sensitivity to pain by impacting mu opioid receptors, thereby raising the pain threshold. This can lower pain perception and reduce physical symptoms.

Grateful people tend to have healthier lifestyles and are more likely to take care of their health. All of these factors, combined with the benefits of positive emotion and optimism, can have a beneficial impact on longevity.

Being able to express and experience gratitude is one of the most empowering ways to connect with the essence of who you are. I call this **soulful gratitude**. Gratitude naturally makes you humbler, while humble people are more grateful, with more capacity for gratitude – these traits are mutually reinforcing. Indeed, a sense of healthy humility can be a great antidote to gratitude deficiency syndrome and sense of entitlement.

Soulful gratitude means connecting with the universe around you, embracing the new possibilities that a spirit of abundance and appreciation brings. Letting go of the untamed ego with all its limitations and its fear-dominant scarcity mindset. Letting go of past regrets and future anxieties with the freedom to simply be more present, right here, right now. Learning to turn the everyday moments in your life into lifelong memories of appreciation. Moving towards service and a sense of greater contribution. In this way, gratitude can become a philosophical emotion, plugging into the bigger picture, letting you see your whole life as a gift.

Gratitude and spirituality tend to be mutually reinforcing. Spiritual people are more likely to feel interconnected with a strong emotional or spiritual link to others. By contrast, someone who lives by the illusion of self-sufficiency is highly unlikely to experience much gratitude. Furthermore, as you grow and develop your sense of gratitude, you experience a deep sense of flow and real fulfilment, an inner knowing that you are connected with the creative force of the universe.

A terrific way to experience soulful gratitude is to simply close your eyes for a moment or two, and focus on your breath as you inhale and exhale. Appreciate the air that fills your lungs with health-enhancing vitality. Acknowledge this magic of life itself, the miracle of being fully alive right now. Experience your heart beating in the centre of your chest with its energy and vibrancy. Move your awareness outwards to sense what you are seeing, hearing, smelling and touching. As you deepen your sense of appreciation for these simple truths, you become more aware of being an active participant in this journey called life. Seeing things differently, through the eyes of the soul.

Gratitude provides a way back to the essence of who you are. It shines a light on the immutable truth that you are not what you do or have, that you are so much more than that. A reminder that, right here, right now, you have all you need for total fulfilment. Gratitude is a reminder of the potential within you to be an agent for positive change, big and small, in the world. I like to say that gratitude can bring hope in the face of despair, light in the face of darkness and healing in the face of brokenness.

IN MY PRACTICE

Here's another case study for you. Tony had been successful in business for many years, at one time employing more than a hundred people. When the economic crash came in 2009, his construction business struggled. He did everything possible to keep it going. He worked around the clock, sold all his assets, including investments that were now 'under water'. He substantially remortgaged his family home, and survived week to week on a very tight budget. Tony began seeing me during this time. While a 'touch of blood pressure' had initially got him to cross my door, over time, like many longstanding patients, we became friends. More often than not our 'consultations' were long chats.

Tony continued to do his best for a number of years, until he learned one day that his remaining bank debts had been, in his words, 'sold off to the vultures'. He was shocked, as he had been under the impression that his bank would give him more time, especially as the economy had begun to recover. Having started the business from scratch 30 years earlier, Tony took this very personally. He felt a failure, and more than anything he experienced a deep sense of shame. He couldn't come to an agreement with the vulture fund and it became crystal clear to Tony that bankruptcy and losing his family home was now inevitable. Tony found this really hard, and for some time was in a dark place.

Throughout that period, I supported Tony holistically on mental, physical and emotional aspects of his wellbeing, and referred him for talk therapy (CBT) with a trained therapist. He read my book *A Prescription for Happiness* and learned some practical tools to navigate the turbulent times he was experiencing, especially the practice of gratitude. I encouraged him to talk about what he was still grateful for in his life and subsequently to express gratitude through the habit of writing down three things each day – WWW (what went well).

Of course, Tony still had so much to be grateful for. While now aged 52, he had good health, his wife was very supportive and he had four lovely children. His entrepreneurial spirit, while badly bruised, remained unbroken. He was, as I regularly reminded him, young enough to start again. Which is exactly what he did. That was five years ago. I'm delighted to say that Tony has had the resilience to rebuild his life and even managed to buy a small home for his family. In Tony's words, 'My gratitude practice became the bedrock on which I found my way back and rebuilt my life. It didn't attempt to deny or downplay what had happened but definitely helped me to realise what mattered most and how lucky I still was in the larger scheme of things. Learning to reframe my experience through the lens of gratitude helped me to let go of the past and move forward with a renewed sense of positivity.'

THE GRATITUDE PRESCRIPTION

There is an old saying in the Irish language: *Tús maith leath na hoibre* – 'A good start is half the battle'. Benjamin Franklin spoke about his morning question: 'What good will I do today?'

GLAD is a mnemonic I use to start my day well. This is a written exercise that only takes a few minutes to reset your mind and heart towards abundance and appreciation. Take a few moments to reflect on each of the following questions. The answers can be brief, just a few intentional words that make a difference.

Gratitude: What or who are you grateful for today?

Let go: What can you let go of today? Little niggles, petty resentments, old ideas that no longer serve you?

Appreciation: Who can you appreciate today? Someone who you will intentionally appreciate through an active demonstration of gratitude or kindness.

Dedicated focus: What are you dedicating your time and energy to today? What is your most important project or goal?

The act of kindfulness

Homelessness has become a major problem in recent years. While the causes may be complex, the care needs for those affected remain the same. It can be easy to remain indifferent or simply blame the 'system' (politicians and/or individuals involved). While no one person can end homelessness, it doesn't mean you need to lose your humanity when confronted by it.

Before lockdown, I remember coming out of a coffee shop one day to see a homeless man seated on the ground nearby. I was drawn towards him and was greeted by a warm hello. He didn't ask for anything, but I took a quick detour back inside and brought him coffee and fresh muffins.

As I gave this small token to him, he smiled warmly and said thank you with his eyes. Of course, it wasn't going to change his situation, but at least for a few moments his day became more pleasant. Mine too. Partly because my guilt was assuaged – I felt better for having done something small, having given something to someone in need.

This is the essence of the age-old 'golden rule' – to treat others as you would like to be treated. By keeping your word, honouring your commitments and reaching out to support others, it comes back to you in many different ways. I can testify to the veracity of this golden rule in my own life and in the lives of the many others that I have been privileged to witness and support as a medical doctor.

For me, **kindfulness** – the simple expression of unconditional kindness through your everyday choices and actions without expecting anything in return – is the essence of this golden rule. Kindfulness in thought cultivates compassion, while kindfulness in word creates confidence. Of course, by its very nature, kindfulness is an action. It's something you do, unlike many other positive emotions which are simply feelings that are experienced. Kindfulness is moving from being self-centred to other-centred, in a spirit of helpfulness. True kindfulness is unconditional and not done out of self-interest or to curry favour.

When you put yourself in other people's shoes and see people as 'other selves' rather than 'others', your sense of purpose and meaning can be enhanced. As an action, kindfulness boosts attentive awareness which builds trust and connection between two parties.

The busyness and, at times, frenetic nature of modern life can discourage people from being kind to others. Many people become consumed by materialism and caught up in their own lives. Furthermore, a scarcity mentality and self-centred notions of entitlement and expectancy can result in kindness being viewed as a sign of weakness rather than strength of character.

I was watching a documentary about the Dead Sea, known for its buoyancy with a salt content so high that anyone can easily float in the water. What's interesting medically is that bathing in the Dead Sea is thought to benefit sufferers from psoriasis. Geographically, the River Jordan flows into the Dead Sea, but nothing flows out of it as it's an inlet, not an outlet. Ironically, there is no life in the Dead Sea. In that respect, it may be considered to be a taker and not a giver, taking all the life and vitality from the River Jordan without giving anything back. Perhaps that's why it's dead – a good metaphor for self-centred entitlement, scarcity mentality and sense of ingratitude.

Hippocrates wrote that a doctor cures sometimes, treats often and comforts always. As a doctor, I believe kindfulness is a key element of more effective engagement with others, enabling better communication and empathic understanding while supporting healing. This is backed up by research showing that when doctors express empathy and kindness during a consultation, their patients' duration of cold symptoms shorten by up to a day[13].

Kindness is a well-recognised character strength and is listed among the commonest reported strengths for many people. In fact, this propensity for kindness is hardwired in your DNA and highlighted by Darwin in his book *Descent of Man* as being a necessary component of evolutionary success.

THE SCIENCE OF KINDFULNESS

Kindfulness stimulates those brain networks that are involved in reward. This happens whether you perform or simply witness a kind act, in person or even online. Furthermore, even thinking about or imagining being kind and compassionate activates the connection and comfort components of the brain's emotional regulation system.

Just as weight training builds your physical muscles, the habit of kindfulness can build the 'compassion muscle' in the brain, enabling you to respond with more empathy to the suffering of others. FMRI scans have also found that feelings of kindness and compassion change the prefrontal cortex. Because of the principle of neuroplasticity, the brain can create new connections as cells that repeatedly fire together wire together. In this way, kindfulness can become a more effortless practice over time.

In terms of the neurobiology of kindfulness (what goes on within the brain itself), it brings about a series of hormonal and neurochemical changes that help to buffer you from stress. Firstly, levels of stress hormones such as cortisol can reduce by more than 20 per cent, reducing feelings of toxic stress, tension or hostility. Secondly, compassion stimulates the vagus nerve, which controls the inflammation reflex and the body's relaxation response, known medically as the parasympathetic nervous system (the yang to the yin of toxic stress). Activating this system helps you recharge from stress. Thirdly, kindfulness enhances positive biochemical responses by increasing the levels of several brain neurochemicals which create feelings of warmth, connection and closeness. These include an increase in DOSE – dopamine, oxytocin, serotonin and endorphins.

○   **Dopamine** increases, because being kind to another

person can light up the brain's pleasure and reward centre the same amount as if you were the recipient of the good deed and not the giver (the 'helper's high').

o **Oxytocin** enhances feelings of trust, empathy and calm. It supports self-esteem and lowers anxiety, providing a natural counterbalance to toxic stress. Oxytocin also supports a stronger immune system and micro-moments of positivity, which are helpful to counteract the busyness and stress of modern living. Hormones like oxytocin make you feel more relaxed and connected to others. Oxytocin reduces inflammation and stress in immune cells and releases nitric oxide, which is cardioprotective, lowering blood pressure and improving heart health. It can also boost endurance by supporting your muscles. Finally, oxytocin, by building connection, makes you far more likely to pay kindness forward.

o **Serotonin** calms you down, supporting feelings of confidence, positivity and happiness. It supports learning, memory and brain function.

o **Endorphins** are natural painkillers, like a micro-shot of morphine, which in addition enable you to feel more calm, energised and optimistic.

BENEFITS OF KINDFULNESS

One of the really interesting things about kindfulness is its threefold impact. Kindfulness impacts, firstly, the doer (the giver), secondly, the recipient of kindfulness and thirdly, the who witnesses the act of kindfulness.

In many respects, giving and receiving are both part of the same universal flow of energy, the yin and yang of life. While you make a living with what you get, you make a life with what you give to others. What goes out to others comes back to you in so many ways. I call this the boomerang effect of kindfulness.

Sense of self: One of the more interesting benefits of kindness is that it's not possible to help someone else without also helping yourself from a health and holistic wellbeing perspective. Kindfulness strengthens your sense of self, supporting self-control, self-worth and self-esteem, simply helping to bring out the best in you. You see yourself as being more caring, compassionate and considerate of others. Kindfulness encourages you to be more open and future-oriented, feeling better and more confident about your own intrinsic good nature. As such, being more kind can be a great way to boost life satisfaction.

Physical health: Research by sociologist Dr Christine Carter – detailed in her book *Raising Happiness* – shows that kindfulness can boost your energy, so you feel stronger, with fewer aches and pains. Kindfulness can be good for your physical health, perhaps because of its impact on your vagus nerve, which influences the body's relaxation response. What I mean by this is that if you want to look after your heart, live more from your heart. Kindfulness can also reduce cognitive impairment in later life and boost longevity. Carter also found that people aged over 55 years of age who volunteer for at least two organisations shows they have a 20–40 per cent reduced likelihood of dying early. This effect of kindfulness on longevity was stronger than exercising four times a week or going to church. Being kind boosts levels of secretory immunoglobulin A, an important immune system antibody. This effect in the immune system is seen whether you are being kind or simply watching kindness – because the immune-boosting benefit is from the result of how kindness feels. By contrast, toxic stress suppresses your immune system irrespective of whether you are experiencing it directly or watching it.

Mental health: Kindfulness can support positive mental health. It can help to build resilience and realistic optimism as protective buffers against toxic stress. It can reduce feelings of anxiety and may have some protective benefits against depression. Kindfulness boosts hope and feelings of being helpful, counteracting the feelings of helplessness and hopelessness that may be seen as part of the spectrum of anxiety and depression. Research in British Columbia whereby highly anxious individuals were asked to do six acts of kindness each week for a month found that they experienced a boost in mood and relationship satisfaction, and socially anxious people showed less social avoidance[14].

Mindset: Kindfulness can boost cognitive performance, focus and attentive awareness. It builds trust as you become a catalyst for positive change. Kindfulness can change your worldview, seeing the world as a more generous and caring place. You can become calmer, less reactive and more responsive. As you develop more perspective, you can see challenges in a more realistic light; better able to see both the wood and the trees!

Emotional vitality: Kindfulness boosts the positivity of your emotional bank account and, as an important human strength, increases subjective wellbeing. Choosing to become kinder and more compassionate can be a great way to feel happier. In a Harvard Business School Survey in 2010 involving more than one hundred countries, societies that were the most financially generous and charitable had the happiest people overall.

Kindfulness can bring on a 'helper's high': an initial feeling of euphoria and positive emotions followed by a longer period of emotional wellbeing and contentment following selfless service to others. It is thought to produce enough endorphins to have the same mental effect as a mild morphine high!

Kindness allows you to feel more grateful and appreciative for what and who you already have in your life, creating an upward spiral of happiness and wellbeing. Knowing you are helping or supporting someone else enhances your own feelings of gratitude. As little as seven consecutive days of kindness can boost your happiness with the degree of uplift in your happiness directly related to the number of kind acts you perform.

Relationships: Kindfulness satisfies a core human need for strong connection. It is a terrific way to boost your relationships as you are perceived as being nicer to be around and seen in a more positive light. It strengthens social ties and sense of community connection, creating more positive social interactions and opportunities to make new friends. In fact, it can be a great way to counter feelings of isolation and loneliness.

At a basic level, choosing kindfulness is acknowledging the humanity of another person by saying to them 'You matter!' Being kinder and more connected to others opens your heart, building empathy, tolerance and compassion. It facilitates shared humanity and fosters humility. Experiencing acts of kindness enables the recipient to feel more appreciated, boosting their self-worth.

In organisations, kindness as a cultural value can boost staff retention and enhance productivity. In fact, choosing to be kind to someone else is a great example of what I call the power of small – how a small gesture of kindness can make a big difference to someone else.

Spiritual vitality: Kindfulness taps into something deep inside of you, a sense of doing the right thing. Through giving people a strong sense that they are doing something that matters, this connects to values, sense of purpose and meaning. Both givers and recipients of kindness can experience a sense of awe when they think about profound acts of kindness or compassion.

THE KINDFULNESS PRESCRIPTION

Elevation is a sense of warmth, expansion, satisfaction, appreciation and affection experienced when you do, receive or observe something kind. You are elevated by witnessing acts of compassion, kindness, moral beauty, courage and loyalty.

This feeling of elevation is one of the reasons why kindfulness is so contagious.

Your commitment to be kinder can inspire others to be kinder and more generous too. Nicholas Christakis and James Fowler, authors of the book *Connected*, found that when one person gives money to others in a game where people have the opportunity to cooperate, the recipients become more likely to give their own money away in future games. This 'learned kindness' habit has been shown to persist in that you don't go back to your former selfish or less kind self.

Similarly, 'pay it forward' is a concept whereby your kindfulness to someone else is returned, not to you, but by that person being kind to someone else, passing it forward like a baton in a relay race. As such, it can create a contagious cascade of cooperation. Research from Stanford has found that one good deed in a crowded area has a domino effect and can improve the day of dozens of people[15]. Perhaps this is one of the best things about kindfulness – how it can cascade through your social networks, creating a chain reaction of positivity (just like an expanding ripple that spreads outwards across a pond when a pebble is thrown in).

In everyday life (pandemic restrictions notwithstanding), suppose that the person you are kind to will interact with and be kinder to on average five other people (first degree). In turn, each of those five people will interact with five others (second degree: 25 people). Each of those people will in turn interact with five more (third degree: 125 people). While these numbers are simply for illustrative purposes, they highlight just how powerful your choosing to express kindfulness can be, positively impacting people you don't even know. Small acts of kindfulness can make a big difference, just as one small pebble can create a big ripple effect in a pond.

Journal

Here are some kindfulness questions to reflect on. Try asking yourself these every day, and they'll help you along the first steps to introducing a conscious practice of kindfulness into your life.

O   Who were you kind to today?

O   Who has been kind to you today? Have you reciprocated?

O   When was the last time you helped someone without expecting anything in return?

O   How can you give more of yourself without expecting anything in return?

O   Who will you be kind to tomorrow?

Here are some ways you can begin.

Random acts of kindness: A random act of kindness (or RAK) is anything that will benefit another person or enhance their wellbeing which involves some input of time or effort by you. Research has found that deliberately doing five RAKs on one day a week over a six-week period can lead to a significant upsurge in your wellbeing[16]. Simply counting your RAKs over the course of a week can boost feelings of gratitude, inner happiness and contentment with a positive relationship between the number of kind acts performed and the level of happiness someone experiences.

When completing these RAKs, there are three A's to remember for yourself: **atunement**, **awareness** and **appreciation**. The key point is that when you do the five random acts of kindness on one single day of the week it makes you more finely attuned to your thoughts, feelings and actions on that particular day. You become more aware of being in the moment in terms of your time and more appreciative of the impact that your words or actions are having not only on other people but on yourself.

Spreading your RAKs over the entire week doesn't seem to work nearly as well, as their positive impact tends to be overshadowed and diluted by everything else that is going on in your life. Research in Spain has found that in an organisation when individuals were split into two groups to either perform or receive acts of kindness, a win-win ensued[17].

o   Those who did RAKs felt happier, with increased job and life satisfaction, less depression and more flourishing.

o   Those who received RAKs were highly likely to pay it forward, creating a ripple effect of kindness throughout the organisation.

My suggestion is to try out this regularly and see how choosing to complete five RAKs once a week can become a new tipping point for your mental health, wellbeing and vitality.

You can use your journal to come up with a list of ideas for these acts; there are so many ways to express kindness and they can be really simple. Consider things that mightn't be part of your daily routine but which can make a real difference. Some ideas include:

○ Donate clothes you haven't worn for over a year.

○ Commit to making a phone call or writing a letter to someone you know who is lonely.

○ Renew contact with an old friend.

○ Donate what you can regularly to a reputable charity.

○ Say something extra kind to someone.

○ Put some spare change to good use by paying for the person behind you at a tollbooth.

○ Do household chores that you normally don't do.

○ Buy the person behind you a coffee when you are in line to get yours.

○ Choose to compliment the first three people you connect with today.

○ Let someone ahead of you in traffic.

○ Send a positively worded text to five people.

○ Be extra patient and considerate as a driver.

○ Help to keep your neighbourhood tidy.

○ Congratulate someone's achievements.

○ Help a stranger.

○ Reach out to someone that you know is going through a tough time.

○ Be a good neighbour.

○ Send someone a handwritten thank you note.

Volunteering acts of kindness: Volunteering your time,

talents or energy to support others can build resilience and self-confidence while helping to fulfil important psychological needs, including the need to feel valued. Such volunteering acts of kindness, or VAKs, tend to keep you outward-looking and other-centred rather than becoming introspective and self-absorbed. It strengthens your sense of interdependence and connection to others – strong factors in enhancing wellbeing.

It gives you the opportunity to build relationships and develop new friendships, to feel more engaged and connected as you face new challenges. Within organisations, volunteering supports a common sense of purpose and enhanced job satisfaction. It enhances a sense of fulfilment and contentment, bringing enriched purpose and meaning to your life.

Loving-kindness meditation: Loving-kindness meditation, also known as *metta bhavana*, is a form of meditation whereby you focus on compassion, loving care, positive emotion and kindness towards yourself and others. It has been found to boost positive effect and reduce negative effect. It may involve the activation of brain areas involved in emotional processing and empathy. In short, compassionate thoughts trigger chemical reactions, which create new brain connections mediated by the vagus nerve and brain neurochemicals including oxytocin.

Research from the University of North Carolina Chapel Hill studied the length of telomeres before and after six weeks of daily meditative practice[18]. Three groups were assigned to either a loving-kindness meditation, a mindfulness meditation or none. In the loving-kindness meditation group, the telomeres did not shorten, highlighting the possibility that feelings of kindness and compassion seem to slow ageing at the genetic level.

Kindness on social media: While social media can allow friends and family to connect and share stories in new ways, it can also be a significant source of toxic stress. Perfectionism, negative comparison, fear of missing out and feelings of inadequacy can all be triggered by social media platforms. The anonymity of being behind a screen can lead some people to be particularly nasty, and their cruel comments can have a really destructive impact. Dealing with the negative mental health consequences of this is something I have seen many times in recent years – and that's why kindness on social media is so important. Remember that there is a human being at the other end of your 'post' button. My own checklist for practising kindfulness online is to think ABC.

o   **Acknowledge** someone who shares a story or vulnerability – let them know you care, even if you don't have any answers.

o   **Be** responsible in what you share and resist the temptation to 'pile in'. Consider the sources and how it may impact others. Rumi cautions: 'Before you speak, let your words pass through three gates.' That is, ask yourself whether if what you are about to say is true, necessary and kind. This philosophy is also appropriate for engagement on social media.

o   **Choose** to be an encourager. When you see something

beautiful or positive in someone, tell them. It may only take a few seconds to say, but for them, those words of encouragement may last a lifetime.

Kindness to self: When kindness is discussed, it is so important to remember to be kind to yourself. After all, you can't pour from an empty cup. The key idea in being kinder to yourself is to understand that you are not a machine; not a human *doing* but a human *being*, defined not by what happens to you but by who you are.

Maya Angelou, the brilliant American poet and writer, put it so well when she said that as you go through life, look at your two hands as a reminder that one hand is to reach out and support others, whereas the second hand is to help yourself. In other words, be kind to others, certainly, but remember to also be kind to yourself. To cut yourself some slack during tough times. It's a similar concept to the thumb on my Hand of Vitality model – remember that as you extend your hand to support others, your thumb points back towards *you*.

Compassion, known as *tsewa* in the Tibetan tradition, is a state of being whereby you extend your relationship with yourself towards others as well. That compassion for others may be considered to be an advanced form of self-interest, where any gap between self-love and love for others simply doesn't exist. To truly care for others, you need to be able to anchor your own sense of self first.

Self-compassion, or being kind to yourself, implies that you start with 'I'. It includes accepting painful thoughts and emotions, your flaws and imperfections. In the culture of perfect online photos, the illusion is created that the perfect, happy life is devoid of painful emotions. Painful emotions shouldn't be so easily medicated away. Helen Keller said: 'Only through the experience of suffering can the soul be strengthened, vision cleared, ambition inspired and success achieved.' Compassion is defined as a deep awareness of the suffering of others along with the desire to relieve it. This requires you, by definition, to have suffered yourself, which builds resilience and deepens your respect for reality. The first of Buddha's Four Noble Truths is the truth of suffering. The thing about suffering is that from an Eastern perspective, suffering and happiness are very much interlinked, in that you can't have one without the other. In the West, we typically resist suffering, repress it or reach for the pill bottle to medicate it away. In Eastern traditions, suffering is recognised as an essential part of the path to enlightenment. Recognising and accepting this inevitability of suffering turns it into a capacity for growth, resilience and enhanced sense of meaning.

Experiencing pain and suffering is a reminder of your limitations, while wisdom gained by reflecting on your experiences leads to a wiser heart. The chances are, you could do with cultivating more self-compassion and overall self-care. Being compassionate towards yourself can become a real game changer for your physical and mental health and overall sense of wellbeing. People with higher levels of self-compassion have higher levels of self-awareness and are more tuned into how they think, feel act and behave. This can enable you to become less reactive and more responsive in your decision-making. Strong levels of self-compassion enable you to take better care of yourself which improves your health, relationships and overall vitality. As you are more self-aware, you will experience lower levels of anxiety and depression.

As you practise self-compassion, you become more relaxed, warm and open with enhanced feelings of trust. Your relationships become more fruitful and meaningful as you experience more personal growth. While some people are naturally very compassionate, it is a highly learnable skill that can be cultivated and developed. Here are four ways to give your self-compassion skills a quick boost:

o   **Physically** – look after your body. Take a walk in the woods, listening to the wind rustling through the leaves or the birds singing. Lie down and listen to some relaxing music. By mindfully focusing on relaxing your physical body, you create small opportunities to feel better with a dose of self-compassion.

o   **Mentally** – mindfully embrace stress and accept painful experiences by cultivating mindful presence. Slow your breathing. Take a pause as you bring your focused awareness onto your breath.

o   **Emotionally** – express gratitude for who you are in your journal. Encourage yourself. Think of how you would encourage a friend facing a challenging or stressful situation. How you would offer kindfulness, empathy, patience, a listening ear, support. Now boost your self-compassion by directing that encouraging supportive talk inwards, towards yourself. What I'm talking about is empowering self-talk, where you accept the reality of where you are and gently encourage yourself to move forward, one step, one day at a time.

- **Spiritually** – write yourself a forgiveness letter. Describe a situation or experience that has caused you pain or suffering. Be objective, don't attach blame. Now reframe that experience through the lens of forgiveness. Forgive yourself for not being perfect, for making a mistake or for simply failing to live up to your ideals. Focus on letting go, learning the lesson and starting again.

Imagine for a moment there was no envy, entitlement or negative comparison in the world. Imagine if everyone ran their own race while supporting and empowering others to do the same. That idealistic vision of the future may be a long way off. But your own future can begin today by choosing to be more kind. Kindfulness is a choice, your choice, to give more to those you meet – even if only the gift of your attention or your smile. Remember, when you choose kindfulness, you can help to make the world a better place – not just your own world, but the world of many others.

The negativity effect

'The negative screams at you, but the positive only whispers.'

BARBARA FREDRICKSON

The adult brain is a fascinating organ, comprising close to three pounds (one point three kilograms) of soft, tofu-like tissue. Fragile too – in fact, extremely so – which is why it is safely encased by the skull bones, out of harm's way. It is made up of more than one hundred thousand kilometres of circuitry, all interconnected by more than one hundred billion nerve cells or neurons. Neurons fire incredibly quickly, perhaps 5 to 50 times per second, with billions of neurons pulsing simultaneously. In the short time it takes you to scratch your nose, billions of brain synapses will have been activated. Each of these neurons has thousands of connections (known as synapses) leading to a vast web of several hundred trillion microprocessors, all wired together.

In the human brain, there are more than 125 trillion synapses in the cerebral cortex alone, which approximates to the number of stars in about 1,500 Milky Way galaxies. That's a huge number, and gives you a sense of the potential – so often untapped – of your brain to influence your everyday decisions and development as a human being.

Although your brain represents about 2 per cent or less of your overall body weight, it is an incredibly energy-intense organ, consuming 20 to 25 per cent of your available energy supply in the form of glucose and oxygen. Just like a computer, your brain is 'always on' – even when you are sleeping – with literally billions of neurons firing each and every minute to keep your body alive and working.

THE SCIENCE OF NEGATIVITY

The architecture and workings of your brain are a timely reminder that despite all the changes in the modern world, on the inside, your brain structure remains the same. The theme of this underlying design and default wiring circuitry remains a bias towards negativity. While feeling positive may temporarily boost your wellbeing, ignoring the negative and not responding to threats can have immediate consequences for your survival, either directly or by disconnection from other people on whom you depend. While there remains much to discover and learn about the human brain, so far, we do know that its architecture has evolved through the development of additional elements to existing structures. In many ways, these resemble a series of interconnected house extensions. Let's take a look at this design.

The basement: the cave

Known as the 'reptilian' or 'lizard' brain, this is the oldest and most basic part of your brain structure. The reptilian brain contains the basal ganglia system as well as the automatic centres that control basic bodily functions such as breathing and temperature regulation. It is also responsible for those automated behaviour patterns that safeguard your survival. In other words, it looks after self-preservation, protection of family and tribe, as well as procreation, referenced sometimes by the four F's – fighting, fleeing, feeding and ... reproducing.

Life in the basement is simply about survival. That's it. There are no home comforts here, no frills or fancy notions. Just living, breathing and surviving. Life in the cave keeps you safe. The reptilian brain recognises what's familiar while allowing you to detect and respond to threats. It operates from the 'better safe than sorry' perspective, and so has a tendency to overreact. Overreacting to a perceived threat keeps you alive for another day, whereas overlooking it might not! Think of a crocodile who perceives a threat – he doesn't call a committee meeting or consider consensus opinion. Snap, crackle and pop. He simply snaps his jaws, cracks his tail and well, the rest is history!

Extension one: the hut
This is the limbic system, the emotional part of your brain, which contains a number of interconnected brain structures responsible for a large degree of your emotional experience. The limbic system operates alongside the basal ganglia to trigger emotional responses to real or perceived dangers or threats. This emotional brain is always on the lookout for the dark cloud behind every silver lining. It includes the hypothalamus, which releases hormones to maintain inner

balance (homeostasis), as well as the hippocampus, which has an important role in learning, memory and spatial reasoning. It contains the ventral tegmentum, important in terms of your motivation, reward and intense emotional reactions to love.

The hut contains dopaminergic neurons involved in the reward system and impulsive behaviour. It also includes the two almond-shaped amygdalae (the red buttons for stress) which help process emotions and attach emotional meaning to your memories. The amygdalae utilise about two-thirds of their neurons to look for threats and, once detected, sound the alarm resulting in the experience or environment being stored in your memory (the hippocampus). This contrasts with positive events, which need to be experienced continuously, in constant awareness, for at least 12 seconds to allow transfer from short-term to long-term memory storage. The amygdalae also regulate emotion, especially in terms of survival (fear, anger, aggression) and support the body to respond to intense emotions of fear and anxiety through activation of the fight or flight response. They also help interpret the emotional content of memories and play a key role in the formation of new memories, especially those in relation to fear.

The hut monitors events both outside and inside your body. For example, facial expressions to determine whether someone is a friend or foe, or to ascertain the presence of negativity or positivity in your environment. If and when the amygdalae perceive a threat, the limbic system is activated to deal with it, with the release of stress hormones from the adrenal gland raising heart rate and blood pressure, readying you for action. As the amygdalae sound more loudly, this leads to death of brain cells in the hippocampus, which calms the amygdalae. In this way, the spiralling effect of chronic toxic stress changes the structure of the brain, making the hut even more sensitive to stress. When the amygdalae are on 'red alert' in a chronically stressed state, the hut impacts other brain areas. These include weakening your self-control and willpower, decreasing your decision-making, reducing your ability to focus and concentrate while increasing your tendency to react, become more irritable and outwardly stressed.

Extension two: the conservatory
This brain area that sits at the front is known as the prefrontal cortex. Think of it as the new conservatory on the old house (the hut with its basement cave). The conservatory is involved with logical thinking, executive brain function and language. While this connects with and has some degree of influence over the amygdalae, the corresponding connections from the amygdalae to the prefrontal cortex are far stronger. This is why it can be so difficult (if not impossible) to simply think your way out of a negative emotion.

Consider your conservatory to be made of fragile glass, which can crack or break easily under the influence of bad weather. Similarly, your thoughts, best-laid plans and intentions can become derailed or side-tracked by distraction and environmental elements around you. This is why you need to triple-glaze the glass in your conservatory with resilience strategies to protect your thinking and enable you to withstand the wind and rain and hailstones. Solar panels on your conservatory enable you to capture the radiant warmth and energy from the sun to your advantage, just as exposure to positivity in your environments, relationships and everyday habits can allow you to think more clearly and creatively with an open, growth-oriented mindset.

Extension three: the smart home

This extension is your mind, and I mention it as a distinct area of its own since, despite all the advances in neuroscience, no one knows where thoughts originate. Consciousness, as this is better termed, exists beyond brain and body. It is also a fact that mind is experienced elsewhere in the body – consider 'gut reaction' and 'heart-based' decisions, for example.

The heart has been long recognised as a focal point for rich emotional experience, spiritual energy and intuitive wisdom. When asked, many people will readily agree they experience gratitude or love more in their heart rather than in their head. Recently it has become apparent that the heart, far from simply being the point of expression of these emotions, is actually able to generate these emotions in and of itself. The heart has a sophisticated nervous system, enabling it to pick up and encode information independently of the 'thinking brain' between your two ears. With every single beat, the heart sends complex information patterns about hormonal, brain and electromagnetic activity that underpin our expression of emotional experience. In other words, the heart can be considered to be a brain independent of the cognitive, thinking brain.

A French proverb says that gratitude is the memory of the heart. The 'heart-brain' is an appropriate term for this epicentre of emotional experience. In fact, I believe it easier to think of mind in terms of having several separate but interconnected components – the heart-brain, gut-brain and conventional thinking brain, as well as consciousness.

The entire nervous system functions as an information gatherer and processor of experience, of emotion, even of thought itself. While all thoughts, images, emotions and sensations require neural brain activity, mind encompasses all of the complexity of the brain and so much more. In fact, conscious awareness of thought and emotion is only the tip of the iceberg of the brain's electrochemical, even quantum, functionality. Mind is not physical, in that you can't measure it; nonetheless, it is very real. While brain can be considered a partial representation of mind, mind is so much more than brain, including consciousness itself.

However, the architectural design and structure of the brain means that you are hardwired for fear, anxiety and survival. This *can* be a good thing. In fact, being hardwired for negativity *is* an adaptive survival tool, an evolutionary hand-me-down from your cave-loving (and cave-living!) ancestors. Inheriting this early warning detection system enables you to detect potential threats in your environment. Just think about the implications of failing to distinguish the lion from the lamb, the angry adversary from the friendly neighbour, the

poisonous berries from the pretty flowers. The bottom line –
being alert to danger, paying attention to threats and taking
action kept you alive back then, and still does to this day. Not
being wrong about threats mattered, and to survive, you had
to win every single day.

As a consequence, negativity (whether emotions, feelings,
events or experiences) affects you more powerfully than
positivity. That's just the way it is! I've found this myself in
my own direct experience. Delivering a wellbeing talk to a
hundred people, my experience has been that many people
find it inspiring and informative, with lots of generally positive
comments afterwards. However, just one person who writes a
negative review can have a long-term impact. Case in point: I
still remember the medic who wrote on a feedback sheet, after
a talk to experienced family doctors more than 10 years ago,
words that are still etched on my brain today – 'Your positivity
makes me sick!' His acerbic comments cut through me like a
knife through butter, while the many compliments received that
day fell away like confetti and were consigned to the memory
scrap heap. Of course, constructive feedback can be invaluable;
a welcome gift in the journey of continuous improvement. But
it is important to keep the impact of negativity bias in check, so
that it doesn't distort your emotional equilibrium, change your
perspective or distort your worldview.

Human negativity bias is a very real phenomenon. The
fundamental 'reality' of your biological hardwiring means that
for most people, despite knowing that they are positive, kind,
loving people on the inside, in their lived reality, the majority

of their time and energy is spent in a state of worry, self-doubt or frustration. While emotions can follow thoughts, most thoughts follow emotions, which is why it can be so futile to encourage someone to think positively without first enabling positive emotions.

Furthermore, toxic emotions and thoughts can become self-reinforcing, leading to a continuous cycle of negativity. As this comes to dominate your inner space, it can drain your emotional bank account and diminish your emotional reserves. Your psychological thermostat becomes set to 'react mode', leading to reduced focus and mental clarity, impairing decision-making and fuelling a cycle of negative stress.

Negativity bias can have a powerful impact on your everyday actions, decisions and relationships. Just think for a moment – when was the last time you thought about a mistake or an insult? Chances are, you can recall some criticism more than a compliment you received. Criticism and bad news weigh more and pack a more powerful punch.

Journal

List the words you associate with positive emotions. Now list the words you associate with negative emotions. Given that the architecture of your brain is designed just like everyone else's, you will likely pay far more attention to negative rather than positive emotions, and find far more ways to describe them as a result.

This is backed up by research by John Cacioppo which

measured brain electrical potential after being shown positive, negative or neutral images[19]. He found that people had a much stronger response in the information-processing part of the brain in the prefrontal cortex after seeing negative images. For pretty much everything, bad is stronger than good. You are more motivated to avoid loss than chance gain. From a very young age, negative information grabs your attention, sticks like Velcro to your memory and impacts your decisions.

First impressions matter: far greater weight is given to negative as opposed to positive words used to describe someone. A bad reputation matters more than a good reputation. A glass may be described as half-full or half-empty. Is it the same thing in many ways? No, not really, especially when it comes to how you interpret this information. If the description of the glass you are given is 'half-empty', then research has found that your view of the glass will be more negative than if it is initially described as being half-full.

Think of 20 things that happened to you today. Perhaps ten of these experiences were positive, nine neutral and one negative. Which one of those things do you remember most vividly? Exposure to negative experiences elicits a stronger response than positive ones do. You will pay more attention to them, generally perceive them to have greater validity, and as a result they become more likely to form the basis for your decisions. Your brain is an A-plus student when it comes to learning from and recalling 'bad experiences', which seep straight into memory. Let's say you have a performance review at work which highlights a couple of areas you can improve in. You feel angry afterwards, unable to let go of the 'negative feedback'. Or you have a blazing row with your partner, after which you find yourself homing in on and magnifying their flaws. Or you have a very good day at work and you have played your role in an important project. You come out of the office to find that your car has been clamped. You eventually get home and feel your day was 'ruined'. All of these are examples of negativity dominance.

In terms of media, because of negativity bias, you will be naturally more attuned to negative news. Whether mainstream or social media, quite simply 'if it bleeds it leads'. This is why it is so important to proactively curate your social media feeds so that you get a disproportionate amount of positivity; ideally, a ratio of at least four to one. Not four to zero, real life is never about denying or suppressing negativity or bad news, just understanding how powerful an impact it can have on your thinking and wellbeing.

Roy Baumeister, who I've already referenced and who is one of the world's leading exponents of willpower and self-control, talks about the 'low bad diet' of ensuring at least four positive news stories for every negative one you entertain. He also describes how media gravitates towards the 'inverse scare law' – the more remote the danger, the more apocalyptic the warnings.

Dan Gilbert, a psychologist, has also described the psychological tendency to become an even harsher critic of how things are, even as things tend to improve, which creates the illusion of no progress. This is a key reason why, despite improvements in almost every conceivable measure of wellbeing, many people are less hopeful now than ever for the future.

Of course, negativity bias is not all bad. Far from it. As well as priming you to avoid danger and take appropriate action, learning to harness negativity for your benefit can improve your decision-making and dissolve destructive thinking patterns. Negativity can sharpen your focus, your drive and your mind. Simply becoming more aware of it can enable you to see the world through less blinkered and biased eyes, better able to control the amygdalae (centre for fear, anxiety and toxic stress), manage impulse control and willpower while making more rational decisions. Awareness brings clarity. Awareness of the piecemeal architecture of your brain, with its hardwired negativity bias, is the starting point to seeing things differently (or at least considering this as a possibility). However, this awareness is very much a logical decision, based on your prefrontal cortex (the conservatory) which, as we know, is subservient to the amygdalae in the emotional part of your brain (the hut).

Which is why, in order to overcome this negativity bias, you need to feel and experience things differently, by building habits to support investment of positivity into your emotional bank account. This is where the ideas and supportive strategies of positive psychology come into their own.

THE BENEFITS OF POSITIVITY

Traditional psychology continues to play an important role

in the diagnosis and treatment of many conditions. It focuses largely on depression and dysfunction – 'what's wrong with you and let's try to fix it' – perhaps improving your subjective wellbeing from a low score (of two, one, even zero out of ten) back to five or six out of ten.

Positive psychology turns this notion of problem solving completely on its head to focus on your strengths, and how you might achieve more happiness and wellbeing rather than simply alleviate suffering. Its founder, Martin Seligman, spent the early days of his career looking at learned helplessness, and its connection with loss of autonomy and depression. He later changed his mindset (and that of the world) by looking at learned optimism, positivity and happiness. Subsequently, he suggested a more encompassing idea of a life well lived, which he termed **flourishing**.

Positive psychology is the scientific study of what makes life worth living: a set of evidence-based tools and strategies that focus on positive thoughts, ideas, emotions and feelings to enhance health and wellbeing. To use the numbers analogy, this means moving you in terms of subjective wellbeing from five to perhaps seven, eight or more out of ten.

As a strength-based approach to living, positive psychology focuses on what's strong as opposed to what's wrong, on what's life-enhancing rather than life-depleting, on building more of the good as opposed to repairing the bad. By changing the way that you look at things, the things you look at start to change. For example, a more positive mindset sees more opportunities, whereas a negative mindset sees more obstacles. It's all about the benefit of small positive changes; how a small extra amount of positivity can create a tipping point that makes you see and experience things differently. Many of the ideas in this book have a strong basis in positive psychology, including reframing, gratitude, kindness, strengths, capitalisation, purpose, optimism, exercise and mindfulness.

Everyone experiences setbacks and has some struggles in life. Everyday stressors like financial burdens, family issues and toxic relationships can all take a significant toll on your energy and wellbeing. There can be a tendency to sweep these issues under the carpet and carry on, regardless of the cost to your wellbeing. Positive psychology can't magically erase these issues, but it can change how you see them. As a result of developing this skillset, you find more meaning in negative experiences, opportunities to learn and grow.

Think about an experience in your past whereby you had an emergency. How did you deal with it? In a cool, calm manner, considering all the options, or by reacting instinctively with your fight or flight response? You are hardwired for these negative emotions: they stick to you like Velcro, whereas positive emotions are transient and bounce off you.

Dealing better with negative emotions means accepting that while negative emotions will always be there, you become more emotionally agile to better process and manage them. You become better able to *respond* as opposed to *react*, building tolerance for distress and bouncing back from negative events. As a result, you become more open to positive experiences in the future.

Broaden and build, as described by eminent psychologist Barbara Fredrickson, is the process of engaging with your positive emotions to broaden awareness and build the resilience to cope better with negative emotions. It implies that negative emotion is real and coexists with positive emotion – one is not a replacement for the other. Broaden and build leads to curiosity, creativity, experimentation and playfulness. In turn this leads to opportunities to build new resources. Positive emotion makes it easier to find the silver lining by detecting positivity in future situations.

In the early part of the twentieth century, *Pollyanna* became a bestselling novel, Broadway hit and blockbuster movie, recounting the story of a young girl, Pollyanna, who goes to live with her (very) miserable aunt. Despite significant adversity, Pollyanna played her 'glad game' whereby she found at least one good thing (a silver lining) in every challenging situation. Even when she lost the use of her legs after an accident, she reframed this adversity through the lens of gratitude (that she was once able to walk). She became so expert at this that her emotional vibe impacted her entire tribe, with attendant positive benefits for many people in the town. While pooh-poohed by many as 'positive thinking', the science behind Pollyannaism is compelling in providing powerful psychological protection against toxic negativity.

As you move away from the fight or flight response, you think more creatively and flexibly, and are more open to new possibilities in terms of what to do next. As your peripheral vision is expanded, your attention span is increased, and you are better able to focus on the big picture. Positive emotions open your heart and mind and expand your outlook on your environment. You broaden your perspective; you are better able to see the wood from the trees. By placing negative emotions within a broader context, you build grit and a sense of realistic optimism. Resilience is enhanced with more coping strategies as you bounce back quicker from adversity. This supports positive mental health as you can build resistance to depression with more ability to see beyond feelings of anxiety or toxic stress.

A **positivity ratio** in excess of three to one is the sweet spot for compounded benefits from positive emotions. In other words, three positive emotions for each negative emotion. This is the ratio for flourishing and while most people have a positivity ratio of about two and a half to one, it isn't quite enough to achieve a tipping point of positivity whereby you can undo the harmful effects of negative emotion. The margins are small in that a ratio of two to one or less is described as 'languishing'. Building your emotional bank account with more positivity enhances feelings of wellbeing and leads to an upward spiral once that tipping point for flourishing is reached.

Positivity can even affect your **heart**. Heart rate variability is a newly described measure of the naturally occurring beat to beat changes in heart rhythm. It is not about lowering the heart rate per se, rather a change in the pattern of the heart rhythm. It enables a mechanism of analysing the heart–brain connection and the stress/relaxation response. If you experience toxic emotions such fear, envy, anger or anxiety, the heart rhythm can become more erratic and disordered, signalling imbalance between the fight/flight (stress) and relaxation response, with a shift towards the stress response.

On the other hand, sustained positive emotions like love, appreciation, hope, interest, joy and compassion are associated with more highly ordered, smoother and coherent heart rhythm patterns as a result of greater balance between the two parts of the autonomic nervous system and a shift towards the relaxation response. This state is called cardiac coherence, which may have several positive impacts throughout the body. First, it can enhance synchronisation between the heart and brain, increasing alpha wave activity in the brain leading to a more chilled out, relaxed state. Second, as the relaxation response kicks in, it seems to fine-tune other bodily systems and functions, including breathing rhythms, blood pressure and gut workings. Third, it can bring on a state of what's known as cardiac resonance, whereby the circulation and cells throughout the body work better and more efficiently. This can improve physical health and, over the longer term, regular episodes of cardiac coherence can positively impact longevity. Cultivating and sustaining a feeling of gratitude and appreciation can lead to more cardiac coherence.

Flow is a universal psychological experience characterised by being effortlessly engaged and energised, coupled with a deep feeling of enjoyment. With the flow experience, you are centred in the present moment, detached from the stresses of the past or future. You are in the zone: peak experience through peak performance.

Many people experience flow from time to time in seemingly simple life situations such as driving the car, cooking, studying, gardening, creative pursuits or satisfying work. Tennis, for example, is a sport in which a state of flow is regularly experienced. There is a clear set of rules that require appropriate responses. The ball must be returned to your opponent's court, giving immediate feedback on the success of your actions. However, when each point ends, no one dwells on the result of the previous point, they merely re-engage with their focus and return to their flow. As you emerge from your state of flow your sense of self is strengthened, boosting self-confidence and self-esteem, knowing that you have overcome challenges with confidence and grace. Creating flow experiences in your life can become a gateway to real inner happiness, a profound tool in the creation of a more productive and rewarding life. As you learn to live in the moment more, you can find flow in the small tasks. Perhaps you even feel it when you are engaged in a conversation with friends. Recognise these moments of flow, where you find yourself in the zone, so you can better channel them into other areas of your life. As the saying goes, flow more to grow more.

IN MY PRACTICE

Take William – another of my patients – for example. William had attended me for years as his addiction to alcohol slowly took hold. Denial is often a key element of the disease, of course, so it took a long time (including a relationship breakdown and repeated work absences leading to a 'last chance saloon' warning from his employer) before William accepted the need for treatment. A short detox regime was followed by 30 days at an addiction treatment centre, with two years of ongoing support. While William had stopped drinking, he still needed to learn the skills of emotional sobriety.

The root of his drinking had been low self-esteem, combined with social anxiety and a tendency to low moods. Alcohol had initially unhinged his ego, resulting in his feeling uninhibited and carefree. However, being a natural depressant, alcohol eventually made his symptoms far worse in a never-ending downward spiral.

The starting point for William's healing was his acceptance of the reality of his situation, which became the bedrock for his eventual recovery. He learned the importance of emotional agility, of not suppressing how he felt or denying negative emotion. Understanding that to experience feelings of anxiety, fear, even anger is part and parcel of being human and a normal part of the totality of life's emotions. At the same time, given their strong potential 'hangover effect', appreciating the critical importance of small, daily investments in his wellbeing to ensure enough positive emotion emerged into his day-today experience. These micro-moments of positivity included learning to savour life's little things, such as a great cup of coffee or a walk in nature. Creating engaging experiences and a sense of flow, by rekindling his lifelong love of fishing, helped to bring a steady stream of positivity into his direction. He also learned the important role of supportive relationships, and how having a network to encourage and empower him was so necessary. That was two years ago, and William continues to grow from strength to strength. He has learned to live one day at a time, with everyday micro-moments of positivity that enable him to flourish and live with more vitality.

THE POSITIVITY PRESCRIPTION

Flourishing is a description of wellbeing by Martin Seligman that incorporates five separate interconnected but independently measurable elements. It is an ongoing process of actively paying attention to and taking concrete steps to live the 'good life'. Flourishing includes making a meaningful difference in the world, experiencing positive emotions, pleasure and enjoyment, using your strengths and talents, as well as developing deep relationships. In his 2011 book, *Flourish: A visionary new understanding of happiness and well-being*, Seligman describes these using the acronym PERMA, which stands for Positive emotion, Engagement, Relationships, Meaning and purpose and Accomplishment. Reflect on the questions and prompts below to see whether you can increase your own flourishing.

o Do you experience **positive emotions** – such as gratitude, anticipation, serenity, awe, optimism, enthusiasm – on a daily, weekly or occasional basis? Can you think of ways to bring more of these positive emotions into your life?

o **Engagement** is a process of being completely absorbed in some activity you enjoy and excel at. Can you choose one activity today – whether that's completing a task at work, making lunch for your kids or arranging to meet friends – and fully engage yourself in it?

o Supportive, meaningful **relationships** are a key ingredient to a vital life. Can you identify a relationship that you would like to further in your own life, and make a meaningful effort to arrange face-to-face contact with that person?

o **Meaning and purpose** are often found through connecting to a cause bigger than yourself. Can you think of a cause that you would like to support in whatever way, and commit to a time to do so?

o Do you set and work towards goals consistent with your values? **Accomplishment** generates positive energy, so aim to identify an area of your life where you could track your efforts and work towards self-improvement.

The emotionally agile person doesn't deny or suppress negative emotion. Instead, they embrace it as an essential part of who they are, along with active strategies to deal with it. At the same time, they use every opportunity to cultivate more heartfelt positivity.

Perhaps the most important decision you need to make in your life, as Einstein once wrote, is: do you live in a friendly or hostile universe? If you believe you live in a hostile universe, you will discover that there are lots of ideas to offend you, which will show up in your life. More hostility, envy and unhinged ego, with people wanting to outdo, hurt and destroy each other.

If you believe you live in a friendly universe, you will act accordingly and actively look for evidence to support your worldview. You will experience more love, joy and compassion as you spend more time in a world of more connection, collaboration and contribution.

One of the main criticisms of positive psychology is that it's simply too focused on positivity and downplays the negative. Of course, it is *not* about only or always thinking positive thoughts, which is neither possible nor desirable. Having a distorted view of reality, discounting all negative possibilities and seeing yourself as better than others leads to self-enhancement bias! Irrational exuberance can be as harmful as intense pessimism.

What I'm saying is that it's all about balance, more specifically, a rebalancing away from your inbuilt negativity bias towards more positivity, neither being blinded by or being blind to problems. Understanding that while you are naturally built for negativity bias, you can intentionally overcome this by bringing more micro-moments of positivity into your everyday choices and conversations. As you embrace more positive experiences, you can help rebalance your inbuilt negativity bias and deal more constructively with negative emotion. As they say in Tibet: if you take care of the minutes each day, the years will take care of themselves. What is the most important minute of your life? This is the idea of small, positive incremental change; the opportunity to rewire your perspective, reframe your outlook and reap the rewards from life with more vitality. There's a Buddhist quote that looks at the same idea: 'Drop by drop is the water pot filled. Likewise, the wise man, gathering it little by little, fills himself with good.'

The Body of Vitality

The focus of this section is to encourage you to value health as a priceless gift while becoming a more active participant in your own wellbeing. Embrace the foundations of physical health in terms of restorative sleep, regular movement and exercise, and nourishing food choices that support your metabolism and microbiome. Look and feel better as health-promoting genes take centre stage. Boost your immune system, which will leave you better able to fight inflammation and accelerated ageing.

Sleep: a natural vitality pill

'There is a time for many words, and there is also a time for sleep.'

HOMER

magine you wake up to read headlines about a mysterious new pill just released to the marketplace. Extensively tested over many years and found to be extremely safe with no adverse effects. With a body of scientific evidence supporting its claims of multiple benefits for your health – a springboard for overall vitality. Something you can take at night (when tired or worn out) and wake up the following morning recharged. Transforming how you feel, with more energy and a brighter mood. Boosting learning, memory and willpower. Helping to better regulate your appetite and manage your metabolism. Reducing your tendency to comfort eat. Lowering inflammation in the body and consequently reducing the risks of heart disease, stroke, diabetes and even long-term dementia. Boosting focus and attention span, reducing feelings of depression and anxiety, while boosting your emotional bank account with more positivity. Strengthening your immune system to fight colds and viruses more effectively. Gifting you vitality-boosting properties that slow down biological ageing.

Perhaps best of all, this 'vitality pill' is freely available without any need for a medical prescription. It's called restorative sleep. Of sufficient quality and quantity, of course, to enable all those promised health benefits to be delivered right to your inbox.

Far from being simple downtime or a time of rest, sleep is recognised as a time of rich creativity and cognitive enhancement. Not only does sleep provide complex chemical rebalancing and an effective clearing system for brain debris; it allows consolidation and enrichment of learning and memory. Overall sleep becomes a catalyst for restoration, recharge and rich renewal.

As Benjamin Franklin was known to say, 'Early to bed and early to rise, makes a man healthy, wealthy and wise.' Such words of wisdom, yet nowadays many people are skimping on sleep and simply not getting enough to support their health and wellbeing. My Uncle Brendan, considered 'a wise owl' as a family doctor, used to repeatedly say about sleep that 'an hour before midnight was worth two hours afterwards'. As we learn more about the science of sleep, what wisdom his words of advice have turned out to be!

Unfortunately, that wisdom was far removed from the reality of my life as a young doctor, where the cultural norm was sleep deprivation. This requirement to forgo sleep and its attendant exhaustion was a simple fact of life. This somewhat sadomasochistic attitude to sleep which implies that 'less is more' still pervades many workplaces nowadays with sleep often seen as being counter-cultural to the goals of productivity and success, particularly in the corporate world. In fact, sleep deprivation has traditionally enjoyed an almost cult-like status, symbolising to many a warrior-like sense of strength and superior productivity.

You may have plenty of reasons to justify this – the deluge of emails in your inbox, demands from online meetings across time zones, or downtime distraction from Netflix or social media. Perhaps simply the everyday challenges of being a working parent of small children.

But the flipside of sleep deprivation is reduced alertness and ability to focus. While that Americano may perk you up and support repetitive, rule-based tasks, it won't help you with tasks that require higher-level creative thinking. Short-changing your sleep is simply mortgaging the potential of tomorrow for short-termism today.

Back in ancestral times, you woke at dawn and went to bed at dusk, a pattern closely attuned to your internal body clock. This simple approach to sleep has really captured my attention in recent years as I see more and more people whose health is being damaged by disrupted sleep patterns.

With the twenty-four-hour culture of bright lights (and, more recently, the explosion of addiction to mobile devices), many people find themselves immersed in environments that are always 'on'. From shift work, time-pressured environments and long commute times, to air conditioning, screens and social media, your environment increasingly mitigates against a healthy sleep pattern. Not to mention daily caffeine consumption, late nights and alcohol. You are ever more distracted with less and less real downtime, unable to recharge from all the 'noise'.

Neuroscientist and sleep researcher Matthew Walker notes in his book *Why We Sleep* that the brain begins to fail after 16 hours of being awake. Ten days of six hours' sleep a night can impair performance as much as no sleep for 24 hours straight. The heavy price you can pay for this is not just your sleep quality (and quantity) but your health and vitality as well.

What about you – do you get enough sleep? Do you wake up feeling refreshed? Do you binge sleep at weekends or on days off? Do you spend time every evening looking at LED-powered phone screens or tablets placed only inches or feet from your eyes?

If you are getting insufficient sleep, then you're not alone. While the World Health Organization (WHO) recommends eight hours per night for adults, research suggests that about two-thirds of adults fail to get this amount, averaging just under seven hours a night. In fact, one in five or 20 per cent get less than six hours' sleep a night with significant adverse effects on their wellbeing[20]. The prevalence of people getting insufficient sleep has exploded over the last few decades. A tiny minority, thought to be less than one per cent of the population, have a genetic predisposition to 'short sleep' and can function adequately on less than six hours a night. While this may be you, the odds are certainly not in your favour!

THE SCIENCE OF SLEEP

Each sleep cycle, from dozing to dreaming, lasts about 90 minutes and almost everyone needs five sleep cycles per night (seven and a half to eight hours). During a sleep cycle, you pass through four separate stages.

○ **Stage 1:** Light sleep, dozing, easily roused. This is the best stage to spend a nap in and why napping for longer than 20–30 minutes leads to residual grogginess as you will have passed into deeper sleep.

○ **Stage 2:** Deeper sleep with a reduction in core body temperature which signals restorative processes taking place in the body. These include clearing out all the debris and broken bits of protein and DNA which have accumulated throughout the day.

○ **Stage 3:** This is the deepest stage of sleep (slow-wave, delta sleep). Waking up here leads to feelings of disorientation.

○ **Stage 4:** This is known as REM sleep, characterised by rapid eye movement. This is where dreaming and emotional processing occurs, extinguishing fear and anxiety. Waking up here makes you more likely to remember your dream.

Science suggests several separate systems that synergistically act on the body throughout the day to influence wakefulness and sleepiness. First, there is your internal body clock, known as homeostasis, influenced by the body's internal cues. At a very basic level, the longer you are awake, the sleepier you will become. Adenosine and waste products accumulate in the brain over time, which increase 'sleep pressure' and increase your desire to sleep. As a result, your brain generally starts to fail when you have been awake for longer than 16 hours.

Second, your circadian rhythm – which comes from the Latin *circa* (around) and *dies* (day) – which is influenced by the light-dark cycle. This allows alignment of the workings of the body over a twenty-four-hour period. Regulated by the suprachiasmatic nucleus in the brain, it is influenced by fluctuations in hormones such as melatonin and exposure to natural (and/or artificial) light. Thousands of years ago, at sunset, this master clock of the brain told the pineal gland to release massive amounts of the sleep-inducing hormone melatonin. This signalled to the brain and body that darkness and the wind-down for sleep had arrived.

Third, there are in addition some very complex neural networks in the brain that interact to turn on or turn off the 'sleep switch'. For example, the ventrolateral preoptic nucleus promotes sleep, whereas other excitatory centres in the brain, including the reticular activating system, promote wakefulness.

Once asleep, the brain remains very active throughout the sleep process. In fact, there is a significant increase in brain blood flow seen during sleep (perhaps as much as 25 per cent during non-REM and at least 70 per cent during REM sleep).

While there is still so much about sleep scientifically that remains to be understood, it is now appreciated that getting enough quality sleep is of critical importance for rest, renewal and recharge.

THE BENEFITS OF SLEEP

Sleep is fundamental to how you focus, function and feel on a daily basis. Awareness of this is a great starting point to prioritising a restorative sleep habit. Rather than wondering about the health benefits of sleep, perhaps it is better to ask if there is any aspect of your wellbeing that sleep doesn't improve. It really can be that powerful an elixir for your vitality. The notion that sleep provides so many health benefits makes complete sense if you think about it, given that it is a daily ritual that has persisted throughout evolution. Your ancestors intuitively understood these benefits of restorative sleep and now, in the twenty-first century, scientists are shining a new light of understanding on this emergent gem for vitality.

Sleep quality can determine how well you fight infection or cope with stress, how creative and decisive you are, even how much you eat! Simply put, to improve your physical health and support your immune system, to support more positive mental health and to enhance your memory and learning: give yourself more sleep. So, let's have a closer look at how sleep really does connect and contribute to each and every aspect of your health and vitality.

Physical impact: Lack of sleep raises stress hormones such as cortisol which narrow blood vessels causing blood pressure to rise. Furthermore, growth hormone (normally produced at night during slow-wave sleep and which can repair blood vessels damaged by cortisol) is reduced with sleep deprivation so that the natural counterbalancing mechanism to cortisol is undermined. As a consequence, you spend your days marinating in more cortisol, resulting in an ongoing 'fight or flight' state with a number of adverse effects on your physical vitality. Every component of your wellbeing can be affected; no system is spared. Little wonder that chronic lack of sleep is likely to shorten your health span and life expectancy.

During sleep, heart rate and blood pressure normally decrease as you dampen down the sympathetic nervous system (stress response) and ramp up the parasympathetic nervous system (rest and digest, pause and plan, recharge from stress response).

Poor sleep increases inflammatory markers, such as interleukin 6, which increase the risks of atherosclerosis and coronary artery disease.

Many studies correlate less than six hours a night of sleep with a significantly increased lifetime risk of heart attack, perhaps up to 200 per cent higher for middle-aged men aged over 45 years of age who get less than six compared to eight hours sleep a night.

Poor sleep quality and quantity are associated with an increased risk of high blood pressure, irregularities of the heartbeat (arrhythmias) including atrial fibrillation, as well as more heart disease and stroke.

Chronic sleep deprivation is now recognised as a significant factor in the development of type two diabetes. Even one week of distorted sleep can affect blood sugar levels and trigger 'prediabetes', whereby fasting blood sugars are elevated.

Each March in the Western world, daylight saving time results in millions of people losing an hour's sleep as the clocks move forward. There is a significant spike in heart attacks and road traffic accidents on the day following this. By contrast, in autumn when the clocks move backwards and people gain an hour of sleep, heart attack rates and road traffic accidents drop significantly the day afterwards.

Lack of sleep also significantly impacts the immune system. First, more inflammatory cytokines are produced, which increase the risk of heart disease and insulin resistance (which can lead to diabetes). Second, the antibody response following exposure to infection is reduced, increasing your risk of developing clinical infection. For example, research has found that if a person is sleep-deprived, flu vaccination may result in production of 50 per cent fewer antibodies.

Third, lack of sleep depletes natural killer cells, leading to increased risk of viral infections. (One night of four hours' sleep may reduce circulating levels of natural killer cells by as much as 70 per cent.)

Sleep deprivation leads to an imbalance in the levels of several brain hormones. Ghrelin levels increase, which make you feel hungrier and seek out more food. You say to yourself, 'I'm still hungry.' Leptin levels, which normally signal 'I'm full', decrease, so you feel more inclined to keep eating and feel less satisfied when full. Endocannabinoid levels increase, which can give you an attack of the 'munchies' (just like cannabis). Sleep deprivation leads on average to cravings for at least 300 extra carbohydrate-rich calories the following day[21].

Spending your day marinating in more cortisol weakens your willpower and self-control, while triggering more insulin release, resulting in a tendency to feel hungrier and store more fat.

Furthermore, lack of sleep is thought to slow fat loss during dieting with a tendency to selectively lose muscle instead. Similarly, muscle performance is affected by lack of sleep with lowered stamina, less time before exhaustion and an increased risk of injuries.

Mind matters: Restorative sleep is a powerful form of neurological recharge for the brain. During non-REM (NREM) sleep, the glymphatic system within the brain shrinks by up to 60 per cent, allowing the cerebrospinal fluid (CSF – the fluid that bathes the brain) to clear out the 'brain trash'. This clear-out includes stress molecules, broken bits of protein, DNA, amyloid, beta and tau proteins that accumulate throughout the day. The glymphatics remove these waste products and neurotoxic chemicals while also playing a role in delivering non-waste products (such as amino acids, glucose and lipids) throughout the brain. A useful analogy is to imagine squeezing a sponge to clear out brain circuits, all while you sleep. If you are sleep-deprived, this sponge effect doesn't do its work as effectively and this can result in memory impairment.

Sleeping provides a highly effective filtering and filing mechanism for memories. It boosts and consolidates learning by moving short-term memories stored in the hippocampus to be filed on a long-term basis in the neocortex. This frees up the hippocampus to learn more without becoming short-circuited and overloaded.

Sleep can also help you to declutter your brain by forgetting less useful memories, for example, what you had for breakfast on the first day of last month. Furthermore, if you are sleep-deprived, the brain finds it much more difficult to assimilate new information. While you are asleep, your brain continues to process data and information acquired during the day. In addition, through the process of neuroplasticity, you form new brain connections that further build and consolidate your memories. Your subconscious mind continues to actively work on finding new insights or solutions to challenges or problems, right through the night as you sleep. It appears that declarative memory (for example, remembering factual matters, such as the capital of Ireland is Dublin) is supported by deep sleep, whereas non-declarative memory (for example, learning to serve in tennis) is supported by REM sleep.

Drowsy driving accidents are common and on the rise because of a phenomenon known as 'microsleeps'. This is where a momentary lapse in concentration for a few brief seconds can be the difference between life and death. Usually seen in people who routinely get less than seven hours' sleep a night, the phenomenon arises when the brain temporarily shuts off from the outside world, with potentially devastating consequences.

Lack of sleep increases levels of stress hormones like cortisol and adrenaline which result in feelings of anxiety and toxic stress. You become more distracted and distractible with reduced focus and attention span and impaired decision-making. With a narrowed sense of perspective, you become more prone to react negatively to your environment and experiences, which can impact your productivity and performance. Overall, you are less resilient, with weakened willpower and sense of self-control.

There is no doubt that improving sleep can be a great investment to support positive mental health. Going to sleep early may provide some protective benefits against major depression, while sleep deprivation may precipitate or unmask some mental health conditions. Feelings of aggression and other behavioural problems can also be triggered. Without the benefits of a good night's sleep, you pay the price in terms of your overall wellbeing.

Emotional and spiritual: The amygdalae are the emotional alarm in the brain (the red button) and are hardwired for fear, negativity and survival. Normally, there is a finely tuned, balancing mechanism between the rational thinking brain (prefrontal cortex) and the amygdalae which stops your fears and anxieties from running away with you.

When sleep-deprived, this fine-tuning between the logical and emotional parts of your brain becomes impaired. The 'noise' from the amygdalae becomes a lot louder, resulting in you feeling more stressed, fearful and anxious. Your emotional bank account becomes depleted of positivity as you become emotionally more negative and reactive. You become less grateful, and more self-absorbed, less likely to experience empathy and compassion, less responsive and more reactive to stress. Instead of 'why not', when sleep-deprived, you are far more likely to say 'why bother'!

Furthermore, an area of the brain near the amygdalae called the striatum (associated with impulsive decision-making) becomes hyperactive when sleep-deprived, resulting in you being more likely to give in to impulsive whims and desires. Emotional mood swings and impulsivity can spell real trouble for addictive behaviours, increasing relapse rates from addiction.

When sleep-deprived, your short-fused amygdalae lack appreciation for nature, higher order thinking or goodness in general. They're only interested in the nuts and bolts of survival. This is a great pity, because you deprive yourself of the possibilities of creativity. Creativity is normally boosted during REM sleep when you are dreaming. Sleep deprivation interferes with the calibration of these emotional circuits. Indeed, one of the most amazing benefits of being in the presence of nature is to enter a flow state whereby you shut off your inner critic, release positivity hormones and move your brain waves to a chilled out, alpha, relaxed state where you can think, feel and be at your creative best. In short, you are less able to disconnect from the noise of the world and to reconnect with feelings of awe, inspiration or transcendence.

The Japanese have a term *inemuri*, which can be translated to mean 'asleep while present'. Sleep deprivation has resulted in an epidemic of presenteeism, whereby people are physically present at work but functionally impaired and far less productive. Ironically, sleep deprivation can result in a form of perceptual blindness, or, as I've heard it said, 'The lights are on but nobody's at home!' As you perceive your lived reality inside your head, your brain just can't appreciate the impact lack of sleep has when you are sleep-deprived.

While many people try to compensate for sleep deprivation with weekend catch-ups and regular pick-me-ups from caffeine, this simply masks the problems that lack of sleep is creating for your overall vitality. Indeed, research has found that three full nights of recovery sleep (more than a weekend) can be insufficient to restore performance back to your usual level after a week of short sleeping. Furthermore, many people in the Western world work night shifts with significant consequences for their sleep patterns and an increased risk of long-term disability.

IN MY PRACTICE

A couple of months back, I had a patient called Annie who attended me as part of her workplace wellness programme, and she admitted that she had been feeling tired and increasingly irritable for some time. A common enough presentation in general practice, with a long list of possible causes. Routine blood work with her own GP had already eliminated anaemia (iron or vitamin b12 deficiency), inflammation, thyroid problems and diabetes before I saw her. Straight away, we homed in on her everyday lifestyle. Sluggish exercise habits, with a tendency to crave sugary carbohydrates (especially at night), along with a poor sleep pattern.

It turned out that Annie hadn't slept well for years, finding it difficult to get to sleep with several awakenings throughout the night. To compensate for this, she was drinking lots of coffee 'to keep me going' and often a glass or two of wine at night to 'relax and chill out'.

Despite her relatively young age of 31, Annie held a senior position at a large tech company where late-night emails were the norm. Furthermore, she brought her phone to bed where she indulged her late-night habit of scrolling through social media.

Once Annie understood more about the science of sleep, and how her current poor sleep habits were sabotaging not just her short-term wellbeing but her long-term health, she was keen to make some changes.

We started with a scheduled 'wind-down' at night with no technology for 90 minutes before bed. This allowed her a 'brain break' from work-related busyness and eliminated late-night blue light exposure with all its deleterious consequences. Given the long half-life of caffeine, her coffee habit was restricted to mornings only, with decaffeinated and green tea recommended options for later in the day. Alcohol was eliminated except for special occasions. After a couple of weeks, Annie began to feel better. She no longer experienced episodes of exhaustion where she felt she was running on empty. She felt her mood was brighter and her willpower was stronger. I encouraged Annie to further improve her sleep habit with a regular exercise programme (though not late at night) and plenty of restorative walks in nature, especially at the weekends. Annie now sleeps much better than before. She can still have the odd night when her sleep isn't great, especially when extra busy at work. Annie has started a mindful meditation practise to help here. Having learned to prioritise her sleep, the result for Annie includes more reserves of energy, more resilience and a richer emotional bank account of positivity. In short, by seeing sleep as something to support her wellbeing, she is now much better able to think, feel and live closer to her creative best each and every day.

THE SLEEP PRESCRIPTION

According to the American Academy of Sleep Medicine, you need at least seven and perhaps up to nine hours of sleep a night. That's a wide range, of course; to determine the amount of sleep you personally function best on, an interesting question to ask is whether you wake up naturally refreshed each morning without an alarm clock. If so, then you are likely to be getting enough restorative sleep. As a medical doctor, I often see people with sleep issues and insomnia. While there are many variables to a good night's sleep, there are a few recurring patterns I see as a doctor that I believe can really make a difference to the quality of your night's sleep. Here are some strategies that I recommend to support a healthier sleeping pattern.

Having a **regular bedtime and rise time** can pay real dividends. Sleeping in at the weekend won't fully make up for lack of sleep during the week *and* will make it harder to wake up Monday morning. As a suggestion, keep an alarm not just for wake up but as a nightly reminder of wind-down and bedtime. Exercise is a terrific habit for physical and psychological fitness and promotes a healthy sleep pattern. Exercise can increase overall sleep time and increase slow-wave sleep. However, it is best avoided within two to three hours of bedtime as the biochemical energy boost from all those lovely endorphins may keep you awake.

Worry and stress can keep many people awake at night, which is why having an effective wind-down ritual is so important for restorative sleep. Defend the hour or two before you go to sleep with a **relaxing routine** that gives you a chance to properly unwind. Gift yourself this time to properly relax and wind-down, completely free from work, for at least two hours before bed. This process of progressive relaxation may include good conversation, reading, watching some comedy or a nice bath, but avoids blue light from digital devices.

In addition to providing relaxation and a mental wind-down, a warm bath at night results in rapid heat loss from the skin surface. This cools core body temperature afterwards which leads to melatonin release, supporting faster initiation of sleep. Try adding in Epsom salts rich in magnesium to further relax your muscles.

Journaling can also help. Writing your 'to do' list for the following day before going to bed can release pent-up worry and anxiety, increasing the quality of your night's sleep. What went well today? Writing down three things at night you feel grateful for, even small things that went well that day, is a wonderful nightly habit to focus on abundance and appreciation, moving you from stress towards a rest and recharge state.

Don't dismiss **naps**, either. Culturally, the siesta is a non-negotiable part of the day for many Spaniards. A short nap of 15 to 20 minutes' duration can be a great, if impractical, habit for restorative recharge during the day. Of course, longer than 20 minutes' duration can result in brain fog and grogginess when you wake up as you enter deeper stages of sleep. Naps are best avoided after 4 p.m., to prevent interfering with your night-time sleep pattern.

If you **can't sleep** after more than 30 minutes in bed or if you feel anxious or worried, get up and read or do some relaxing activity until you feel sleepy. Of course, persistent worry and anxiety that interferes with sleep may indicate an underlying chemical imbalance, anxiety disorder or depression and it is important to discuss this with your primary care physician if of concern.

Create an environment conducive to sleep. Keep your bedroom as **dark and cool** as possible. Optimal bedroom temperature for sleep is cooler than many realise, at 65 degrees Fahrenheit or just over 18 degrees Celsius. Ensure your sleeping surface (pillow and mattress) are comfortable. Keep digital devices out of your bedroom and your alarm clock out of view to avoid clock watching.

The problem with technology and sleep is twofold. Firstly, all that information and noise late at night keeps your brain on a **high alert** awake state, making a mental unwind and slowdown far more difficult. Secondly, as a highly visual creature (with about a third of the brain dealing with visual information), the master clock in your brain is exquisitely sensitive to the blue wavelength light from your digital device. This is the key reason why using mobile devices in the evening impacts sleep onset. The blue wavelength light fools the brain into believing that the sun has not yet set. As a result, your internal body clock is wound back by two to three hours. In addition, melatonin release is delayed by several hours, so it takes longer to get to sleep. The amount of melatonin released is reduced so that sleep quality is affected, including less REM sleep (so important to extinguish feelings of fear, anxiety and toxic stress). As a result, you feel a lot less rested and more drowsy the next day. This so-called 'digital hangover' effect can last for several days after exposure. Therefore, avoid blue wavelength light for at least two hours before bed.

Natural light exposure during the day for at least 30 minutes helps to regulate sleep patterns by enhancing energy and shutting off daytime melatonin. Even cloudy days provide a light intensity of 10,000 lux (compared to only 250–500 lux indoors). Consider walk and talk meetings at work as a strategy to get outside. Morning time is best for blue light exposure which helps to optimise your internal body clock.

Ideally, **avoid eating or drinking** within three hours of bedtime (except for water or herbal, caffeine-free teas). While light snacks may be okay, heavier meals definitely affect sleep quality. Drinks late at night can also result in frequent trips to the bathroom, impacting sleep quality. In general, foods low in fibre and high in processed carbohydrates, salt and saturated fat can all adversely impact sleep quality.

On the other hand, certain foods provide the brain with **essential nutrients** that support a more restful night's sleep. For more restful sleep, think fibre-rich foods such as those found in a Mediterranean diet, protein-rich foods, potassium and natural melatonin sources. As a natural relaxant, magnesium deactivates adrenaline, promotes feelings of calm and can support sounder sleep. Magnesium also supports gamma-aminobutyric acid (GABA), an important brain neurotransmitter that supports sleep. Magnesium deficiency can lead to insomnia. Foods rich in magnesium include spinach, bananas, brown rice, nuts and avocado.

Watch the **coffee**; it (and to a lesser extent tea) is rich in caffeine, which is an adenosine receptor antagonist. This means it blocks adenosine, a brain substance that enables you to get to sleep. Caffeine can reduce total sleep time, increase time to fall asleep, reduce sleep efficiency and worsen perceived sleep quality. It reduces deep sleep and increases arousal. Caffeine can take eight hours to wear off, so mid and late afternoon coffee can certainly keep you awake at night. In fact, the half-life of caffeine is four to six hours, meaning that 300 milligrams of caffeine in your 11 o'clock Americano may result in approximately 75 milligrams of caffeine circulating in your blood 12 hours later. You don't have to be a maths genius to figure out why too much coffee can keep you awake! Furthermore, some people are extremely sensitive to the stimulant effects of caffeine. Genetic factors play a role here and older adults may be more sensitive to its effects. While I love to savour and enjoy a cup or two of really good coffee, I suggest avoiding caffeine in the second half of the day. If you have difficulty sleeping, cutting it out for a while can be very helpful.

In terms of **alcohol**, less is definitely more! Alcohol is a sedative drug and will anaesthetise your brain, reducing REM sleep and deep restorative sleep. By keeping you in the lighter stages of sleep, it can lead to frequent awakenings, especially when the alcohol wears off in the middle of the night. Initially, it sedates the prefrontal cortex (the seat of reasoning and reason) – the part of the brain which influences and controls your behaviour. As it is relaxed by alcohol, you tend to loosen up and become more extroverted. Alcohol then progressively sedates other parts of the brain. The result is that, rather than falling asleep, you tend to become anaesthetised with your brain frozen in stage two sleep. As a result, you don't get the deep restorative sleep that you need, with resultant fatigue the following day. Furthermore, your sleep tends to be fragmented with frequent awakenings that you don't tend to remember. After a few alcoholic drinks, you lose out on REM sleep, leading to more feelings of anxiety and toxic stress the following day. Alcohol also generates break-down products called aldehydes, which interfere with REM sleep, as well as the building and consolidation of memory, which may continue for several nights after learning.

If you **snore**, you may have a form of sleep apnoea which affects sleep quality and is often associated with high blood pressure. There are many other medical conditions which may impact sleep, including anxiety, depression, prostate issues, chronic pain and other conditions, as well as breathing issues. Discuss your medications with your doctor to see if they affect sleep. Many prescription medicines can impact sleep, including treatments for heart and blood pressure, steroids and antidepressants (SSRIs), over-the-counter decongestants (for coughs and colds) and allergy medicines such as antihistamines.

Sleeping tablets are a sticking plaster solution for those who are experiencing difficulty with their sleep. As well as physical tolerance, dependence and addiction issues (on top of psychological dependence) they can increase the risk of falls and overall mortality. They cause relative daytime sedation, which can increase caffeine consumption, which in turn negatively impacts sleep in a virtuous cycle. In my opinion, they are best avoided.

Some people with sleep issues have low levels of **melatonin**. This is perhaps why melatonin supplements have become popular recently to support sleep in several conditions, particularly in those who suffer from jet lag as well as shift workers with varied daily work patterns.

Melatonin appears to work by reducing the length of time it takes to fall asleep. Of course, it can cause side effects, so if you are considering melatonin for sleep purposes, make sure you talk to your doctor first to ensure this is a suitable option for you.

Several randomised control trials have shown the benefits of **mindfulness** on sleep quality. Mindfulness simply moves you away from the stress state towards the relaxation response of the parasympathetic nervous system.

Consider counselling in the form of **cognitive behavioural therapy (CBT)** from a trained therapist if you have ongoing sleep issues. Talk therapy can be highly effective as a support strategy to improve your sleep pattern.

Mindful movement

'It is exercise alone that supports the spirits, and keeps the mind in vigour.'

CICERO

I magine something that can provide immediate benefits for your brain and body. Lower feelings of stress and tension. Help to clear any brain fog and let you think more clearly, boosting memory and motivation. Feel more positive, supporting your health and vitality. Welcome to exercise and movement, perhaps the greatest self-care gifts you can give yourself.

As the first doctor in modern times to establish the link between physical exercise and the prevention of heart disease, diabetes and depression, Jerry Morris is my hero. In the UK, after World War II, it was noted that unprecedented numbers of people were suffering fatal heart attacks.

Morris began his research and first noticed a significant difference in the heart disease rates of London bus drivers and bus conductors, despite the fact that both groups were cigarette smokers.

The drivers, who spent about 90 per cent of their working time sitting down, had significantly more (about twice as many!) heart attacks as the conductors (who typically climbed about 750 steps collecting fares throughout their working day).

While these results were compelling, Morris wanted more evidence, so he continued his research with two other groups. Firstly with postmen, where he found that those postmen who delivered mail either by bicycle or on foot had far fewer heart attacks than those who spent their working time sedentary and seated at desks. Finally, he researched the activity levels of civil servants during their time off. Those that partook in vigorous exercise had lower rates of heart disease than those who didn't. His overall finding for all groups was that the reduction in heart attack rates was simply related to how active you were and was independent of either weight or waist size.

Morris's pioneering work was published in *The Lancet* in 1953, at a time when exercise was considered by many physicians to be harmful to health. So much so that if you were living in a two-story house, your doctor may well have advised you at the time to move to a bungalow to minimise strain on your heart! A lifelong exerciser himself, Jerry Morris led by example, working and exercising until his death at the age of 99. In 1996, he was awarded the first international Olympic medal in exercise sciences for his work in recognising this link between exercise and heart disease.

Thousands of years earlier, your 'hunter-gatherer' ancestor may have moved up to 14 miles a day in search of food. In those days of feast or famine, movement was essential for survival. Over time your ancestor's prefrontal cortex grew and evolved to make them smarter and sharper. As a result, your brain's biological blueprint is hardwired to move regularly by your genetics, metabolism and to keep your brain and body in peak condition. Quite simply, your genetic make-up is geared for exercise and movement.

The problem nowadays is the serious mismatch between this biological blueprint and basic lifestyle habits that exist for many people. Many people are physically inactive, with more time than ever spent sitting at the desk or sofa, stockpiling unused calories as surplus fat stores.

THE BENEFITS OF MOVEMENT

Movement matters, big time! Sedentary behaviour is defined as not actively exercising for 30 minutes per day, three days in a row, for three months straight. The American Medical Association describes this as an independent risk factor for heart disease. Being sedentary may be far more deadly than being obese, a fact that's beginning to garner serious attention. Sitting slows down (and eventually shuts off) biological systems that break down fats and sugars, moving you towards fat storage, and a pro-inflammatory, accelerated ageing state. In addition, when sitting, less feel-good hormones and neurotransmitters flow to the brain which impacts negatively on mood.

Even women who exercise regularly may increase their risk of dying prematurely by up to 37 per cent by sitting for more than six hours a day (versus those who sit for less than three hours a day)[22]. Sitting time becomes an independent risk factor for mortality, regardless of time spent exercising.

In fact, studies have found that, compared to those who sit for less than three hours a day and are most active, being less physically active and sitting for more than six hours a day increases early death by 48 per cent in men and 94 per cent in women.

A study of more than 30,000 women in the USA and published in the *American Journal of Preventive Medicine* found that sitting for more than nine hours in total a day increased depression rates[23]. Research has linked prolonged sitting with an increased risk of a number of adverse health conditions, including obesity, diabetes, heart disease and metabolic syndrome (a cluster of conditions that includes raised blood pressure, high blood sugar, excess body fat around the waist, raised triglycerides (blood fat) and low levels of HDL (good) cholesterol).

While the headlines proclaim that sitting is the new smoking, scratch beneath the surface and you will find that this statement is only partly true. You see, smoking any amount of cigarettes is bad for your health. There is no lower safe limit of cigarette consumption. Even being in the presence of someone who smokes exposes you to all that toxic sidestream smoke, and it has been rightly banned from workplaces. No one would ever suggest banning sitting from the workplace or that being in the presence of someone who is sitting down could be bad for your health. Of course not, because there's nothing wrong with sitting down (once you're in a good ergonomically adjusted chair) – just don't sit down for too long. Because, if you do, some research suggests that it may increase your risk of early death from all causes just as much as smoking cigarettes does.

Research looked at people who spent more than four hours a day in front of the TV or other recreational screen time, and compared against those people who spent less than two hours a day. There was more than a hundred per cent increased risk of cardiac events (including heart attack and chest pain) and almost 50 per cent increased risk of death from any cause in the group that spent longer sitting looking at screens[24]. What's important to note is that this was an independent increase in risk that was separate to whether these people had other risk factors for heart disease such as smoking, high blood pressure, etc.

The bottom line is that prolonged sitting is bad for your health. Not just in front of the TV or digital device – any form of extended sitting, whether at work or driving, can be harmful. Furthermore, moderately intense exercise at the gym or elsewhere doesn't appear to significantly offset the risk posed by prolonged sitting. In other words, prolonged sitting is an independent risk factor for adverse health conditions, no matter how healthy the rest of your lifestyle may be.

Exercise can be a great **antidote to feelings of anxiety**. In many ways, it is like an 'anti-anxiety vaccine', supporting you in feeling calmer and more centred. Aerobic exercise programmes such as running, cycling or swimming and especially high-intensity interval (HIIT) training can be particularly helpful and may have the added benefit of also reducing your body's sensitivity to feelings of anxiety. Brain circuits are rewired with regular exercise, so that the tendency of the amygdalae to overreact to perceived danger is dampened down. Resilience is enhanced as you realise you have more control over how you feel, and that you can choose to face your fears and worries with more confidence.

Exercising regularly helps you to feel better about yourself, boosting your **mood and self-esteem**. As you feel and look better, exercise can encourage a more positive self-image, boosting self-belief and self-worth. Taking positive action in this way is a key element in building a more confident version of you. This confidence will likely spill over into other areas of your life, supporting you to work towards other important goals.

As the brain's reward chemical, dopamine is released in response to any form of reward, whether pleasurable or painful – including likes on Facebook, alcohol, sugar, shopping, drugs or gambling. Dopamine is released from an area of the brain called the nucleus accumbens, which tricks the brain into believing that those rewards are needed to survive. This pathway is hardwired into the brain as an automatic response pattern. Dopamine release is one of the key mechanisms in the brain pathways for addiction and dependency on the craving initiating it. While the prefrontal cortex tends to inhibit behaviours that may result in harm, it doesn't fully develop until you are in your mid-twenties, which is why teenage drug exposure can be so dangerous in terms of addictive potential. The good news is that exercise can support **recovery from addiction** by creating an effective form of distraction, enabling you to deprioritise cravings. It may also dampen down parts of the brain involved in the addictive process. Because exercise is a natural antidote to feelings of toxic stress, anxiety and depression, it helps to fill the void created by the loss of the addiction, while building self-confidence in your ability to change for the better.

At a basic survival level, movement boosts learning, enabling you to find food as well as figuring out where it was last time. Food then becomes fuel to support further **movement and learning**. Exercise can help protect the brain against age-related loss of cells from the hippocampus, an important part of the brain for memory and learning. Exercise increases a process known as autophagy which removes toxic substances from inside your cells, especially those in your brain, making you smarter at any age. During exercise, diffusion of blood flow away from the prefrontal cortex can make it difficult to learn complex tasks. However, immediately afterwards, your brain can be sharper and more focused. This is why an important idea-creation session in the afternoon may well benefit from a lunchtime workout. Quite simply, the fitter you are, the sharper your brain functions will become.

Research from Australia has found that regular exercise is probably the most effective form of **willpower support and self-control** available[25]. By monitoring self-regulation over a several-month period while participating in a regular exercise programme, it was found that self-regulation and willpower can be developed or depleted, just like a muscle.

Furthermore, they discovered a domino impact of exercise on other health-enhancing habits. As participants increased their numbers of visits to the gym, they began to eat more healthily, smoked and drank less, lost their tempers less often, curbed impulses such as overspending, procrastinated less and kept more appointments. They even left their dishes in the sink less often! In many ways, exercise can be considered a miracle drug for willpower, so exercising regularly will make you even more motivated to keep going!

Some **stress** certainly can be good (essential even), in order to grow, learn and thrive in the world. However, toxic stress can be seriously bad for your health and may shorten telomeres, particularly if you are sedentary and stressed. Research has found that exercise buffers the effects of stress on your telomeres[26], with perhaps as little as 14 minutes of exercise daily protecting against stress-induced shortening. Exercise enables your brain and body to adapt and respond rather than simply react to stressful challenges or threats. As such, exercise can be a terrific natural stress buster, enabling you to destress and blow off steam. As a low-level form of stress itself, regular exercise elevates the stress threshold, buffering you against life's other stressors. Exercise reduces the levels of your body's natural stress hormones, such as cortisol and adrenaline. The rush of cortisol initially boosts brain-derived neurotrophic factor (BDNF), brain learning and readies you for 'fight or flight'. As a result, you feel less stressed, embrace stress and cope with life's challenges more effectively. Regular exercise builds a protective buffer and raises the tipping point for the 'fight or flight' stress response to be triggered. How much exercise and movement do you need? The more stress you have, the more you need to move (in addition to other self-care strategies) to prevent the damaging effects of marinating in all that cortisol.

Exercise changes your concept of 'self' and can be a highly effective **antidepressant**, and just as effective as prescribed pills. It doesn't simply impact solitary chemicals or molecules the way medication tends to. As a natural, brain-boosting antidepressant, exercise recalibrates the signalling pattern in the entire brain. In the first SMILE study (Standard Medical Intervention and Long-term Exercise), sufferers from depression were placed into three separate groups and assigned treatment for 16 weeks with either medication or aerobic exercise or both. There were 156 older adult participants, who were randomised to four months of either aerobic exercise, sertraline at dosage consistent with standard clinical treatment of depression, or a combined exercise and sertraline regimen. The exercise prescribed involved 30 minutes three times a week, at 70 to 85 per cent intensity, with a 15-minute cool-down period afterwards. The results found about a 50 per cent improvement in each group. However, 10 months later, the exercisers had far lower levels of relapse compared to the medication or combined group (8 versus 38 per cent). Furthermore, those people who reported regular exercise at this stage were more than 50 per cent less likely to be depressed, regardless of initial type of treatment. A follow-up study also included a placebo group and home exercisers (to control for the potential social interaction benefits of exercising in groups). Results found that exercisers and medicators did better than the placebo group. One year later, taking regular exercise was the only significant protective factor against relapse risk. Therefore, the SMILE study shows just how effective exercise can be for depression in terms of treatment and preventing relapse.

The word 'emotion' is spelled **e + motion**, a reminder that exercise and motion (movement) leads to (positive) emotion. Just a few minutes of movement can change your emotional state for the better. A major review in 2018 of more than 500,000 people, varying in age from teenagers to twilight years, found that taking physical exercise correlates strongly to feelings of happiness[27]. Instead of trying to think your way out of toxic moods or thoughts, *move* your way instead towards more emotional calm and mental clarity. Furthermore, exercise and movement may provide a protective buffer from varying degrees of emotional stress, meaning that you tend to be less fazed by stressful situations if you have just exercised. Aerobic, strength and flexibility exercises are all effective as ways to boost emotional positivity and feelings of happiness. Small increments of exercise – perhaps as little as 10 minutes – can have a big impact on mood and enable you to express a better version of you in the world. This positivity can spill over into every aspect of your life, improving your relationships, career and overall enjoyment of life. The impact of small extra amounts of movement in your day can really add up. I call this the 'X factor' of exercise, how bringing forth a collection of activity-induced brain chemicals can boost feelings of happiness and contentment, enabling you to think, feel and be closer to your creative best. Exercise can also bring on the 'flow state' whereby you are in the zone of peak experience and peak performance.

At any age, exercise and movement can begin to switch on the **epigenetic machinery** to enhance positive health changes. For a start, it's a tremendous way to feel fitter and stay younger looking. It is better to be physically fit and overweight than of normal weight and inactive. Regular exercise increases the number of mitochondria (the powerhouses) in your cells, which gives you an energy and vitality boost while building your endurance and stamina, so you can quite simply do more. Exercise boosts your metabolism, turning your body into more of a fat-burning machine, supporting weight control and helping to detoxify the body from stored carcinogenic toxins. More importantly, exercise improves body composition.

Regular exercise greatly **reduces the risk of disease**, particularly of heart attack and stroke, even for those who already have heart disease. It strengthens your heart muscle, lowers blood pressure and tends to thin the blood by increasing a process known as fibrinolysis (breaking up clots). Exercise helps lower total cholesterol levels, raise the HDL (good) cholesterol level and lower the LDL (bad) cholesterol level, while helping lower the blood fat (triglycerides) level. As well as increasing insulin sensitivity and reducing the risk of developing diabetes, regular exercise significantly reduces the risk of complications in people with existing diabetes. Exercise can reduce the risk of developing several types of cancer and lower your risk of getting gallstones. Exercise can also boost the immune system, building more resistance to colds and flus.

Regular exercise **aids sleep**. It can help to reboot and restore your natural circadian rhythm and body clock, enabling you to hit the hay and sleep more soundly. However, it is best to avoid heavy exercise late at night, as this can leave you too buzzed up to sleep!

Regular exercise can help spark up your **sex life**, protecting men against erectile dysfunction and helping women with arousal. Regular exercise helps to reduce cellular inflammation and lengthen your health span (the number of years you stay healthy for). Telomeres may lengthen with regular exercise, which can lower biological age and support healthier ageing.

THE SCIENCE OF EXERCISE

Regular exercise has been shown to be a powerful ally for your mental health and psychological fitness. While it is really good to talk, movement and exercise can be just as good (sometimes even better) in terms of boosting brain function.

Research has found that exercise increases the growth of new brain cells in several key areas. Firstly, in the hippocampus (located in the temporal lobes), which improves learning and long-term memory. Secondly, in the prefrontal cortex (the brain's CEO), the area involved in executive functioning, including planning, organising, learning from mistakes, initiating or delaying a response, consequence evaluation, focus, attention and working memory.

By increasing blood flow to the brain, exercise supports the creation of new pathways between brain cells in these areas (hippocampus and prefrontal cortex) through a process known as neuroplasticity. This helps your brain's memory (in terms of learning and retaining new information) and supports your IQ as you become smarter and sharper.

Furthermore, these brain areas most improved by exercise (the hippocampus and prefrontal cortex) are the brain areas most susceptible to neurodegenerative disease and age-related neurological decline. While exercise can't necessarily prevent dementia, the brain-boosting benefits in these areas can maximise the chance that it takes far longer to take effect.

In terms of exercise and mental health, there's a collection of 'feel-good' brain chemicals, enhanced by exercise, that I call the 'Magnificent Seven'. These stimulate the chemical reactions in your brain to create a more positive mental and emotional state. These brain chemicals work together to fire up positivity and finely tune brain circuitry and activity. Furthermore, they play a major role in buffering the impact of toxic stress, anxiety and depression on the brain. Exercise plays a key role in boosting, balancing and fine-tuning these Magnificent Seven.

Let's get to know them in more detail:

○ **Serotonin:** In many ways, serotonin acts as the brain's own natural antidepressant. Sometimes known as the 'policeperson of the brain', as it controls other brain chemicals, serotonin affects mood, aggression and impulsivity. It brings a sense of calm, safety and security, while enhancing feelings of positivity and happiness. More recently, the microbiome – the bugs in your gut – has been found to produce a significant amount of the body's serotonin, adding new understanding to the term 'gut–brain connection'. Perhaps exercise may also boost this mechanism of serotonin production.

○ **Endorphins and endocannabinoids:** Exercise stimulates a number of pain-reducing and positivity-producing chemicals, including brain endorphins, a kind of natural painkiller that can help you to feel calm, optimistic and energised, creating a pleasant, even mildly euphoric feeling after a moderate workout. Endocannabinoids are biochemical substances similar to cannabis that are produced naturally by the body. Their levels increase with exercise when they can easily cross the blood–brain barrier to produce their anxiety-reducing and mood-calming effects.

○ **Noradrenaline:** Exercise also increases levels of noradrenaline, a chemical that can work in moderating the response of the brain to toxic stress and dampen down feelings of anxiety.

○ **Dopamine:** Exercise promotes the release of dopamine, which boosts motivation, attention, learning, reward and satisfaction. As a result, you are more likely to persist with a new habit and to be more motivated to get out in the world and do things, which, of course, leads to a greater sense of personal accomplishment. Exercise also helps counteract the perceived lack of challenge and associated reduction in dopamine levels as you get older.

○ **GABA:** This is an inhibitory brain neurotransmitter whose main job is to reduce or block the activity of nerve cells in your nervous system. It helps your brain to disengage from 'fight and flight', thereby reducing stress and supporting relaxation. It also plays a role in balancing between calming alpha brainwaves and busy beta brainwaves. As such, GABA creates calmness, alleviates anxiety and stress, while soothing your brain, supporting a more restful night's sleep. It builds resilience to threats, both immediate and longer term.

○ **Oxytocin:** Sometimes known as the 'tend and befriend' hormone. It plays a role in the regulation of your emotional responses and boosts feelings of trust, empathy, caring and compassion. As a pro-social hormone, it supports positive communication and a willingness to reach out and connect with others. At the same time, it can reduce levels of stress hormones and feelings of hostility or helplessness.

As you can see, when you push your body with physical exertion, all sorts of good things start to happen. Firstly, you begin to **burn fat** which increases levels of tryptophan in the bloodstream. This crosses the blood–brain barrier to enhance the production of serotonin, dopamine and noradrenaline (all part of the Magnificent Seven). This enhances attentive focus, awareness, motivation, patience and optimism.

Secondly, the heart produces **Atrial Natriuretic Peptide (ANP)** in the atria as the heart beats faster and levels of this increase further with increases in heart rate. ANP travels from the heart to the hypothalamus in the brain where it seems to dampen down the sympathetic nervous system and put a brake on the stress (fight or flight) response. By reducing feelings of anxiety and toxic stress, ANP has an overall positive benefit, enabling you to feel calmer and more relaxed after a moderate workout. Research in Germany has found that if ANP is blocked from getting into the brain, one hundred per cent of the participants got a panic attack[28].

Thirdly, exercise and HIIT in particular, fires the brain cells, which release a substance called **brain-derived neurotrophic factor (BDNF)**. This is part of a family of neurotrophic factors which builds brain cells and supports critical circuits between thought, emotion and activity. It is believed to help with learning, higher thinking and decision-making. Described as 'miracle-grow' for the brain, it supports brain plasticity and synaptic growth of new brain cells. It acts like a reset button on stress, protecting the brain while helping to repair and replace brain cells. This development of new brain cells is known as neurogenesis and occurs in the brain's learning centre (the hippocampus), which is involved in creating and retrieving memories. BDNF protects brain cells against the corrosive effects of cortisol in areas that affect your mood, including the hippocampus. Overall, BDNF keeps your brain cells younger and more robust, while supporting brain plasticity as the nerve cells branch out and connect with each other in new ways, forming new interconnected patterns. This boosts learning and memory, building new brain cells and helping to protect them against memory loss or cognitive decline as you get older. Furthermore, BDNF and serotonin enhance the action of each other in an upward spiral. Doing a better job on the job!

Fourthly, **adrenaline** is released through exercise, which boosts learning and enables you to learn from a stressful situation. While chronic stress is corrosive and damaging to the brain, the brain is buffered from this through the release of BDNF. This restores brain cells and raises the bar to future stress episodes by strengthening brain circuits. Movement and exercise result in microscopic muscle fibre breakdown which must be repaired. This dynamic process involves growth factors which repair muscle and cross into the brain across the blood–brain barrier to support neurogenesis, create new brain cells and cement learning.

IN MY PRACTICE

This brings me to another of my real-life patients. When I first met Mary and looked at the long list of medications she was taking, I had that sinking feeling that many doctors can relate to when it comes to polypharmacy. So much medication, where to even start? At that time, Mary's chronic pain syndrome had overtaken every aspect of her life. What had initially started out as a lumbar disc issue many years earlier had progressed to chronic pain from a combination of degenerative back and neck arthritis, as well as soft tissue inflammation. A serious road traffic accident 15 years ago, resulting in several fractures, had certainly made things worse. She had seen various medical specialists down through the years and had availed of procedures from therapeutic facet joint injections to various nerve blocks. Still, her pain continued and she had ended up on a plethora of long-term painkillers including anti-inflammatories, codeine-based preparations and twice-weekly morphine patches. The pain negatively impacted her mood, of course, which had led to various antidepressants being prescribed. Her overall quality of life was not good.

Had she tried exercise to help? I explained how exercise and movement can release natural pain-killing endorphins which may very well be of some benefit to her. Furthermore, the boost in positivity neurochemicals was likely to boost her mood. She gave me a sceptical look as I quickly explained that I knew some people who were doing tai chi (a very gentle form of rhythmic movement). Would she give it a try, if her sister, whom I knew, would agree to go with her?

Mary tried the tai chi. Three months later, she said she was really enjoying it. Next, she started aqua aerobic classes, and the next time I saw her after that, she was ready to discuss reducing her medication. Great news, I thought, having previously highlighted some of their downsides. Over the next six months, Mary increased both the frequency and intensity of her exercise routine, while in tandem she slowly reduced her dose of painkillers. Each day involved either swimming, tai chi or yoga. In addition, she found she was able to walk much more easily and regularly went for 30- to 40-minute walks with her friends.

Mary still has pain today – some days, she says, are better than others – but she feels she has much more control over her pain symptoms now. Apart from a tablet for nerve pain which she takes at night, she is now more likely to have an Epsom salt bath than to take prescription painkillers but will take two paracetamol when she really needs to.

While clearly not a panacea for all cases, Mary's story is a real-life example of just how beneficial a regular movement and exercise programme can be. Furthermore, Mary feels fitter and more alive than she has done for many years. Her mood is better than it has been for years, and she finds herself looking forward to things again. Over this time, Mary has become stronger, with better balance and a more upright posture – all key elements for healthier ageing.

For many of us, just Mary, a positive change is to simply move more. I call it mindful movement: making movement the default position throughout your day.

THE MOVEMENT PRESCRIPTION

A question I'm often asked is 'How much exercise should I take?' Of course, the answer depends on so many factors, including:

○ What are your exercise and health goals?
○ What is your existing level of fitness?
○ What is your existing schedule like?

One of the key ideas in 'lifestyle as medicine' is that the amount of exercise and movement you take is a new vital sign for your health and wellbeing. I've believed for years that exercise is the greatest pill of all. Now lifestyle medicine considers your exercise habits to be as important as your blood pressure or weight. In other words, it is a new vital sign as a marker of your wellbeing. Furthermore, it has been shown to be as good as at least 10 medications in terms of its health benefits. Lifestyle medicine guidelines for exercise have evolved from research involving thousands of studies. As a general rule, in terms of exercise and movement, here is the latest 'prescription' for exercise as medicine. Consider the mnemonic **FITT**: that is, **frequency** of exercise, **intensity** of exercise, **time** spent on exercise and **type** of exercise. In terms of this exercise prescription, I define success as taking enough exercise and movement to optimise the epigenetic expression of your genetic potential.

I've put together some areas below that can be considered as support strategies to incorporate more exercise and movement into your routine.

Get sweaty: When you push yourself and sweat that little bit, the heart beats faster and improves oxygen consumption in the body. You release more BDNF, boosting memory and sharpening your focus to literally become a sweaty genius. Build some moderately intense exercise into your lifestyle (you can talk but not sing during it). Examples would include jogging, cycling, tennis, even brisk walking. Aim for at least 150 minutes over the week.

More vigorous exercise (you can't talk or sing during it) for 75 minutes per week is an alternative to 150 minutes of moderately intense exercise. HIIT involves alternating periods of regular intensity with short, sharp bursts of high intensity whereby you go flat out for periods of perhaps 30 to 60 seconds' duration. It can be done with many different types of exercise, including a cross trainer, running, exercise bike, etc. There are huge benefits in terms of time efficiency and minimising the risk of overtraining, but of course, HIIT is not for everyone, and if you're not used to this type of training your body will quickly let you know! It places big demands on your heart, so start slowly and build up gradually, having got the go-ahead in advance from your doctor.

Stay strong: Lean muscle mass is now considered to be one of the leading biomarkers for healthy ageing. Building lean muscle mass is one of the best ways to boost metabolism and stay biologically younger. Strength training burns fat and builds muscle, which will burn more calories, keeping your muscles and bones strong and healthy. Two or three fifteen-minute sessions, spaced out during the week, utilising the main muscle groups are ideal. Many people are unaware that strong muscles also lead to strong bones, which can help minimise the risk of fracture due to osteoporosis. Numerous studies have shown that strength training can play a role in slowing bone loss, resulting in stronger, denser bones. Furthermore, strength training targets bones of the hips, spine and wrists, which are the sites most likely to fracture. Other benefits include reduced risk of high blood pressure, better balance, less functional decline with ageing and less fat and weight gain. You're never too late to reap the benefits either. Even centenarians can build muscle strength!

Just move: Hippocrates said, 'If you are in a bad mood go for a walk. If you are still in a bad mood, go for another walk.' Do you find that, like me, you do your best thinking while walking? Now, I love to get out in nature and spend time walking in the Mount Congreve gardens close to my home here in Ireland, so much so I call it my 'creative laboratory'. Moving outdoors in nature, what I call 'green exercise', can boost feelings of calm and connection which move you away from the stressed state towards a state of deeper relaxation. Even a short walk outdoors can enhance creative thinking. In addition, more movement can have a positive domino impact, motivating you to move more often, eat better and take better care of yourself. In many ways, movement can be a keystone habit for your health and vitality. Research published in the *British Journal of Sports Medicine* in 2018 suggests that substantial fitness benefits accrue from walking at a pace of at least one hundred steps per minute.

Here are a few ideas to get you started.

o   Stand whenever you have the chance, while on coffee break or talking on the phone.

o   Standing desks enable you to vary your working position and can be ergonomically ideal as well.

o   'Twalk' (walk and talk) your way to better health, boost thinking and develop more creative ideas. Why sit down for an hour's meeting if you can walk for part or all of it instead?

o   Adhere to the 30-minute rule – I believe that ideally you should stand up every 30 minutes or so and walk around. I also talk about the 50-minute hour; by that I mean stand and move for 10 minutes each hour.

○   Set an alarm reminder every 30 minutes to stand up, stretch or stroll for a glass of water.

○   Design your environments to encourage movement – use the stairs instead of lifts.

Spiritual exercise: Exercise as medicine also incorporates a holistic spiritual dimension. This growing appreciation of the mind-body-spirit interface can be seen by the increasing popularity of yoga, Pilates, tai chi and qigong, all of which can have significant benefits for your wellbeing. I include stretching here, as a mindful way to not just relax and unwind but as an important habit to prevent injury and keep the body loose. It is an important part of any exercise programme, and stretching at least twice a week is recommended. Exercises to strengthen the lower back and stomach muscles, often called core stabilisation exercises, are now recognised as being key to injury prevention.

Seek support: Because of both emotional and attitudinal contagion, we are all significantly influenced, in both a positive and negative way, by the people we spend time with. If your friends are couch potatoes who binge on Netflix, chances are that's what you will do too. Conversely, if your friends are into exercise and the outdoor life, that can really support and encourage you in terms of a positive exercise habit. Regular exercise can be a great way to connect with friends in a fun setting, find new friendships and build existing relationships through cultivating shared interests. This is one of the great benefits of joining an exercise class: like-minded people with a similar interest, encouraging and supporting each other, while working out and having fun. Think 'play out' as opposed to 'workout'! Having positive people in your space that can strengthen and support you can be invaluable for your mental health and overall wellbeing.

Plan ahead: Precommit. Design your environment to make it easier to exercise and move more. Consider using a journal to monitor your progress. Recording how you felt before and after exercise can be a powerful motivator to persist and keep going. Write down your exercise goals. How important are they to you? Why? How confident are you in achieving them? Who can support you? What activities do you enjoy or like most? Can you make them part of your schedule and routine? Will you do this alone or as part of a group? Who can act as your accountability partner?

Start simple: Making changes that stick isn't easy. What's the smallest thing you can do today to build a more sustainable exercise habit? It's all about starting! It's never too late to reap the game-changing benefits of exercise, no matter how busy you believe you are, how tired you think you are, or how unfit you may be right now. Self-care requires you to exercise and move. Be sensible, listen to your body. Don't exercise when you're sick, or sore. Stay well hydrated. Be specific. Figure out ways to exercise that support your specific needs right now. For example, if you have back trouble, then swimming, yoga or Pilates can be terrific. If your knees are creaking, then non-weight-bearing exercises such as cycling or an elliptical cross trainer can really help.

And remember, small changes can make a big difference. Every journey of a thousand miles begins with a single step. Taking that first step may be the single best thing you can do to not just feel better but to reap multiple health benefits and slow down potential age-related cognitive decline. Overall, you can face a flourishing future of thriving vitality rather than one of fragile survival. By embracing the health and vitality-inducing benefits of exercise, you can quite literally change your life. Small steps each day towards a healthier, more revitalised version of you.

What are you waiting for?

Mindful eating

Have you ever considered just how much time you spend eating each day? Well, if your habits are 'typical', you may spend about 90 minutes each day eating, with a proportion of that time eating while distracted by driving, watching television or other forms of multitasking. In other words, mindless eating.

There is no doubt that beliefs about food can be wide-ranging, with an endless number of influencers and opinions nowadays about this or that latest 'superfood', etc. Just for a moment, consider the many cultural factors and religious beliefs about food, the role of family traditions and upbringing, health issues and food intolerances, work practices and lifestyle habits. You will begin to appreciate the vast spectrum of sometimes quite entrenched ideas about food that can be hard to change.

Not to mention the punitive nature of the word 'diet' with its implied denial and suffering. Suppose you decide you're never eating crisps or chocolate again. When you're on your 'A game', with high self-control and willpower, the 'never again' rings clearly in your mind. But on a Thursday evening, tired and stressed after a tough day at work, willpower is depleted and now your emotional brain will scream loudly, 'Give me crisps and chocolate, I deserve them.' Whether you believe you do or not is incidental – the point being that negatively framed food choices of giving up this or that are often doomed to failure because of the make-up of your brain with its limited supply of willpower.

Which is why I'm such a fan of positive health changes, particularly the potential impact of small positive changes over time. You eat at least three times a day, which adds up to 1,100 times a year or 11,000 times over the next 10 years. Simply add in one extra portion of vegetables or fruit each day and see how those benefits can compound over time.

Ultimately, the best diet is the one that works best for you, and what's best for you may not be what's best for someone else. Just like your fingerprint, you are unique. The opportunity is in becoming more aware of why you make the food choices you do *and* considering whether choosing differently could lead to a healthier version of you.

THE BENEFITS OF MINDFUL EATING

Mindful eating is being present and aware to the cues that trigger eating behaviour – hunger, boredom and other emotions – as well as those associations and cues that tell you that you have had enough. It is based on the Confucian principle known as *hara hachi bu* – eating until no longer hungry (generally about 80 per cent full) – as opposed to when you are full. Eating mindfully enables you to appreciate how all your senses (touch, sight, smell, hearing and taste) individually and collectively engage with food. You have heightened awareness of the experience of eating and the effects it has on your body. You become more attuned to how your eating habits impact the world around you, enabling you to connect more deeply to nature and with other people.

Mindful eating can support your self-awareness to choose healthier eating behaviours with long-term benefits for your health and wellbeing. Small, positive changes in those daily decisions and habits can have a big impact over time. Mindful eating can also be very helpful in combatting emotional eating and eating to excess.

Heightened awareness of thoughts, feelings, sensations and behaviour in the present moment, as well as eating triggers (including emotional cues), provides a space to allow you to choose to respond differently. As you change your thinking about food, you boost self-control to support a healthier eating pattern. You eat more consistently, less dependent on the vagaries of your willpower muscle, as you better design your environment to support more mindful eating and plan ahead. Heightened awareness provides clarity to respond more mindfully to make healthier choices for you, your family and the planet.

Mindful eating allows for better atunement to your hunger and satiation (full up) signals, a process that takes about 20 minutes. You reduce emotional eating (brought on by stress, sadness, sense of isolation, etc.) and environmental cues to eating. You eat more intentionally as opposed to automatically, and reduce the frequency and severity of binge eating. Chewing your food thoroughly enhances your enjoyment of food as you are better able to engage your senses and explore all of the tastes (sweet, sour, salty, bitter and savoury) on your palate. It enables you to digest your food better which can also support less overeating. This all leads to a more sustainable healthy eating pattern which supports long-term weight control.

It promotes appreciation, enjoyment and savouring of food (from its origins, the people who prepared it, to the food itself) in addition to the opportunity that food provides to satisfy your hunger.

Mindful eating is not a calorie-counting collection of cans or can'ts when it comes to your food choices. Rather, it is your commitment to a more positive engagement and relationship with food. It empowers you to choose healthier eating habits, enabling you to embrace the rich potential of nutritious food. Mindful eating brings the bigger picture into mindful focus, extending to your entire relationship with food, including how you purchase, shop, prepare and cook, as well the environments and people you eat among.

THE SCIENCE OF EATING

Ancel Keys (1904–2004) was an American scientist who became intrigued by the differing degrees of heart disease between countries. This led to his Seven Countries Study and subsequent discovery of the health benefits of the

Mediterranean diet. Having heard from an Italian professor that there was little heart disease in Italy, he decided to take a road trip throughout the Cilento coastal areas of southwest Italy to find out for himself. While on a short stopover for coffee at a small fishing village called Pioppi, he noticed that there appeared to be a lot of elderly people around. Active, energetic and old. Very old indeed. On checking further, he discovered that 81 of the 500 residents at the time were more than 100 years old! Keys did his research. As well as a Mediterranean diet of fresh vegetables, fruit, olive oil and seasonal foods reared locally, he noted their lifestyle included regular movement, a strong sense of connection with community and sustainable living. Rates of heart disease were very low compared to Americans and North Europeans. So impressed was Keys by these findings that he decided to move permanently to Pioppi with his wife Margaret, adopting the Mediterranean diet and local lifestyle. Having authored three books, he went on to live to the ripe old age of 100. Coincidence, or not?

More recently, attention has switched to a similarly sized hamlet located in the Salerno province, about 85 miles from Naples, in the southern Italian area of Cilento. Acciaroli is the name of this village, located just a few kilometres from Pioppi. Here, 10 per cent of the population of 600 people are aged over 100. What's more, rates of heart disease, dementia, diabetes and cataracts are very low. The residents are immersed in the Mediterranean diet, and particularly fond of anchovies, olive oil, herbs (especially rosemary) and wine. Laid back, living life to the full with a smile on their faces, they have a striking sense of joie de vivre and an uncanny ability to stay stress-free.

In terms of health benefits from good nutrition, the Mediterranean approach to eating is the star pupil. Firstly, as a heart-healthy diet, it reduces the risk of heart disease. Research involving 15,000 people from more than 39 countries over four years, published in the *European Heart Journal*, found that close adherence to the Mediterranean diet led to a significantly lower risk of heart disease, stroke or death from ischaemic heart disease[29].

The PREDIMED study in 2013, published in the *New England Journal of Medicine,* looked at 7,000 men and women who had either type two diabetes or were at high risk of heart disease. It found that those who ate a calorie-unrestricted Mediterranean diet (including extra virgin olive oil and nuts) reduced their risk of cardiac events by 30 per cent. Further research on 25,000 men and women published in the *Stroke Journal* found a reduced rate of stroke in women (but not men) who followed the Mediterranean diet (reducing risk of stroke by up to 20 per cent in those with highest risk)[30].

The Mediterranean diet was found, in a four-year follow-up of some participants in the PREDIMED study, to reduce the risk of developing type two diabetes. Other research published in 2013 in the *American Journal of Clinical Nutrition* (a meta-analysis) found the Mediterranean diet helpful for control of blood sugar. It may also reduce the risk of certain cancers, especially colorectal and breast cancers, largely due to the emphasis on whole grains, fruit and vegetables, as well as being rich in antioxidants and anti-inflammatory agents.

In terms of mental health, the Mediterranean diet has been associated with a reduced risk of depression. Four longitudinal studies found that compared to a pro-inflammatory SAD (Standard American Diet), the Mediterranean diet reduced the risk of depression by one-third. Forty-one observational studies, published in *Molecular Psychiatry* in September 2018, found reduced rates of depression in people who lived by the Mediterranean diet.

Finally, the Mediterranean diet as part of an active lifestyle can support longevity. Telomeres are located at the ends of chromosomes and help protect the ends from fraying. As telomeres shorten, rates of chronic disease increase and life expectancy lowers. Research in Harvard University in 2014 (on more than four thousand women), found that greater adherence to the Mediterranean diet was associated with longer telomeres (and that small positive changes in dietary habits can make a big difference).

While the evidence in support of the Mediterranean diet in terms of reducing disease and mortality is significant, it is the overall message that matters most: moderation in portion size, avoiding snacking between meals, restricted eating windows and socialisation of eating patterns. Good food loves company – think family, friends and occasions to enjoy food together. Add in an active lifestyle with regular movement, time to recharge from stress, and a real sense of belonging to engage more fully with the elements of the Mediterranean lifestyle.

So, what's in it?

Consistently regarded as one of the healthiest 'diets' on the planet, it combines traditional foods and cooking techniques, with tremendous flavours from countries that border the Mediterranean Sea. Regarded as a healthy and highly sustainable way of eating by the World Health Organization, it is more a way of life than a diet per se. While the word 'diet' usually implies excluding foods or cutting back, with a plant-based Mediterranean emphasis, the simple idea is that more is better. The Mediterranean diet provides great variety and versatility as well as tremendous health-boosting vitality. As a diet of inclusion rather than exclusion (all food groups included), it remains flexible enough to fit in your particular dietary preferences while avoiding the restrictive feel of many other diets. The focus is on colour and consistency of nutrients as opposed to calories.

Here's my understanding of the Mediterranean diet in terms of positive lifestyle change to support your health and vitality. There is an emphasis on whole foods, meaning foods as close to their natural form as possible (including fruit, vegetables, whole grains, beans, peas, lentils, nuts and seeds). The variety of elements together appear to provide the health benefits rather than a single 'superfood' ingredient as such. Perhaps best of all you don't need to travel further than your local food market or supermarket to bring home these tremendous health-boosting benefits.

Healthy fats: These are a key component of the Mediterranean diet and include monounsaturated and polyunsaturated fats. They reduce LDL and total cholesterol levels, reduce blood fat levels (triglycerides) and raise HDL (good cholesterol). Trans fats are avoided and saturated fat is minimised. A rich source of monounsaturated fat is olive oil, especially extra virgin olive oil, which is less processed and contains more antioxidants. It reduces LDL and total cholesterol. Monounsaturated fat is also found in canola oil, seeds, avocados and tree nuts (almonds, walnuts, pecans, cashews, hazelnuts). Avocados contain oleic acid which lowers LDL cholesterol – avocado oil can also be used in cooking. Polyunsaturated fat is found in nuts and seeds but particularly in oily fish including albacore tuna, salmon, mackerel, sardines and herring. These fats reduce blood fat levels, lower inflammation, reduce risk of clots and reduce growth of cholesterol plaque on blood vessel walls.

Plant- rather than meat-based: Plant-based foods are the building blocks of the Mediterranean diet. A largely plant-based diet (plenty of vegetables and fruit, whole grains, nuts, seeds and plant-based protein sources such as beans, peas, lentils) can significantly lower LDL cholesterol, blood fat and blood pressure. Their high fibre content helps to maintain a healthier body weight as you feel full sooner after eating. Fibre also helps regulate blood sugar levels.

Of course, the high intake of vegetables, fruit and nuts are a rich source of antioxidants, which support telomeres and help protect against chronic disease, age-related degeneration and oxidative stress. Plant-based foods contain thousands of health-boosting phytochemicals and protective factors which support health and longevity.

Fruit and vegetables: Aim for seven to ten servings daily of a rainbow in colour from beetroot and blueberries to red peppers and everything in between. Think variety in flavour and texture.

Wholegrains: Swap in wholegrain bread, pasta and cereal. Think traditional Mediterranean grains like rice (brown, black and red), bulgur, barley and farro. Wholegrains are rich in soluble fibre and are a great swap for refined grains. Oats are rich in soluble fibre which binds to cholesterol in the gut and helps to remove it from the body before it reaches the bloodstream. A bowl of oatmeal or porridge is an easy way to get more soluble fibre (about two grams). Current nutrition guidelines recommend at least 5 to 10 grams of soluble fibre a day out of a total fibre intake of 35 grams.

Nuts and seeds: Heart-healthy nuts include almonds, Brazil nuts and walnuts – all rich in omega-three fats as well as trace elements such as magnesium and zinc. Seeds rich in heart-healthy omega-three fats include flax and chia seeds.

Beans, peas and lentils: These are all rich in soluble fibre, while beans of all shapes and sizes are also rich in health-boosting trace elements such as potassium and magnesium. They are a key component of a heart-healthy diet.

Fatty fish: Eating omega-three-rich fatty fish (sardines, tuna, salmon, mackerel) two to three times a week can help to lower blood fat (triglycerides) and prevent irregular heartbeats. Grill and avoid deep fried. Shellfish including oysters and mussels are included.

Moderate dairy: Yogurt (Greek and plain), kefir and small amounts of cheese are all allowed. Try pecorino cheese (rich in omega-three fats).

Spice it up: Include plenty of fresh herbs and spices. Think rosemary, parsley, garlic, thyme, turmeric and black pepper. Minimise salt.

Liquids: Of course, staying well hydrated by drinking enough water is so important for your metabolism, energy and focus. Remember that approximately two-thirds of the adult human body is made of water. Your brain is more than 70 per cent water, your muscles (including your heart) are over 75 per cent water, your lungs are more than 80 per cent water, your skin is 64 per cent water, and even your bones are 30 per cent water! Water is an essential *nutrient* that your body needs lots of. Drinking enough water to stay properly hydrated means drinking about 3.7 litres per day for men and about 2.7 litres for women

For me, good coffee is one of life's great pleasures, to be savoured. Furthermore, regular coffee intake can reduce the risk of developing several chronic diseases, reduce accidents (perhaps by boosting attention and sense of caution) and support longevity. A major study published in the *European Journal of Epidemiology* in 2019 found an association between the lowest mortality rates and drinking about three and a half cups of coffee a day. Of course, too much caffeine may cause palpitations, trigger anxiety and keep you awake at night given caffeine's long half-life. If coffee's not your thing, consider drinking tea, not just regular tea but green and herbal teas, loaded with antioxidants and health-boosting vitality. As for alcohol, this should be drunk in moderation (think one glass rather than a bottle!).

Desserts: Fresh fruit – again, think rainbow in colours. Keep sweets for special occasions. Dark chocolate (at least 70 per cent and ideally 85 per cent cacao) is rich in resveratrol, which is heart-healthy and good for the circulation, and it can also boost HDL (good cholesterol). It contains theobromine, which translates from Greek as 'food of the gods'.

As I've said throughout, **small changes** can add up over time to make a big impact. Here are a couple of simple, manageable things you can try to make your diet more Mediterranean.

○   Try to eat a rainbow in colour each day (from blueberry and beetroot through to red peppers and everything in between).

○   Try to include more than 30 different plant ingredients in your diet over the course of a week (yes, count them!). For example, if you have a handful of mixed seeds containing flax, chia and sesame seeds, then that counts as three.

○   Dip wholegrain bread in extra virgin olive oil and spread a little hummus on top for three more (hummus from chickpeas, extra virgin olive oil from olives plus the wholegrain bread).

○   Try extra virgin olive oil instead of butter or dairy spreads, dip your wholegrain bread in extra virgin olive oil flavoured with a sprig of rosemary or some garlic, for example.

Your **microbiome** is your unique collection of up to one hundred trillion microbes, consisting of thousands of different species that live throughout your body, mainly in your gut. The health and diversity of your microbiome is now recognised to play an important role in many biological processes and pathways in your body, in your health and disease prevention. These include effects on your mood, metabolism, weight and immune system, as well as absorption of key minerals such as calcium and magnesium.

Dysbiosis – imbalance of your microbiome – can lead to many problems including feeling more tired, stressed and anxious, weight gain, low mood, memory problems, 'brain fog' and inflammation. The modern Western diet, rich in sugar and processed food, is considered toxic to the needs of a healthy microbiome. Other causes of this imbalance or dysbiosis being researched include lack of sleep or exercise, toxic stress and the role of environmental toxins.

Poor sleep, jet lag and shift work also affect the microbiome in a manner that can trigger obesity. As an example, fascinating research has been done whereby faecal matter from jet-lagged individuals was placed in the guts of healthy mice[31]. The mice then become obese, whereas faecal matter from healthy individuals (not jet-lagged or doing shift work) had no impact on the mice.

Clostridium difficile (C. diff) is a severe hospital-acquired infection that can potentially have fatal consequences. Research in the USA has found that transferring faecal material from healthy individuals into the rectum of patients with C. diff by a process known as faecal microbiotal transfer can be curative. All of this research highlights a growing understanding of the pivotal role your microbiome plays in maintaining good health.

The microbiome connects and continually communicates with your brain, influencing your emotions and mood through the production of various neurotransmitters such as serotonin, dopamine, acetylcholine and GABA. A healthy microbiome influences the brain's neurotransmitters to keep the brain perfectly balanced and functioning properly. Take a moment to think about whether your current food choices nourish or neglect your microbiome. There's almost always room for improvement! While many factors can adversely affect it, here are some dietary pointers that can help to rebalance your microbiome.

Prebiotics are essentially fibre-rich foods that the bugs and bacteria in your microbiome feed on. While you are unable to digest fibre because you lack the enzyme required to break it down, microbes living in the colon can break down, ferment and feed on prebiotic foods. This fermentation process releases short-chain fatty acids (SCFAs), which are thought to influence many health-enhancing processes in the body. In addition, these SCFAs lower the pH of the gut environment, which influences the types of gut bacteria that can flourish in this more acidic environment. (For example, it reduces the growth of harmful bacteria such as C. diff.) Prebiotic foods include garlic, onion, Jerusalem artichokes, asparagus, leeks, tomatoes, carrots, seaweed and bananas. Wholegrains such as oats, barley and wheat as well as beans, fruit and vegetables are all good sources, as well as spices including turmeric and cinnamon.

Although lifesaving for severe bacterial infections, the rise of **antibiotic resistance** due to over-usage is a significant cause of concern. Remember that antibiotics will not only knock out harmful bacteria but good bacteria in your microbiome as well. Furthermore, many upper respiratory tract infections are caused by viruses for which antibiotics are completely ineffective. If you do need to take an antibiotic as prescribed by your doctor, be mindful of the benefits of taking plenty of prebiotics and probiotics with it to mitigate against the adverse impact of the antibiotic on your microbiome.

One of the best ways to maintain the health and diversity of your microbiome is to eat a diet with a **wide variety** of plant-based foods. Getting at least 30 plant-based elements into your weekly diet appears from research to improve diversity with a link to better heart health, mental health and weight management. Think whole grains, nuts and beans. A teaspoon of mixed seeds – each seed type counts!

The good bacteria in your gut like to feed on the dietary fibre found in complex carbohydrates (wholegrains), fruits and vegetables. If your diet is lacking in these, then your bugs will feed on the mucosal lining of your gut instead, which may lead to inflammation and potential illness. Appreciating this critical importance of your microbiome can enable you to make better lifestyle choices that can gift you the benefit of more sustainable improvements in your health and vitality.

Brilliant research carried out at the Salk Institute has highlighted just how important the **timing of eating** can be[32]. While the brain's circadian sleep–wake cycle is triggered by exposure to light, every other organ in your body has its own internal clock. Whereas the first light of the day triggers your brain clock, it is the first cup of coffee or morsel of food you have in the morning that turns on these 'organ' body clocks. Hence the case for a restricted eating pattern to enable the cells of your organs enough time to rest, repair and recharge for optimal functioning.

Many people tend to eat over more than a 15-hour time span each day. Do you? Intermittent fasting means that all food is consumed within a maximum time window of 12 hours each day. Outside of this time window, water is allowed, as is herbal tea so long as it doesn't contain any caffeine, milk or sweeteners. In addition, finish eating at least three hours before bedtime to enable the body to slow down for rest, repair and rejuvenation.

Learning from the fruit fly is a key way to understand the genetics of ageing as they share a number of genes with humans and have a life span of 30 days which makes them ideal subjects to study. San Diego University research on fruit flies, published in *Science* in 2015, has found that genes responsible for the body's circadian rhythm play a key role in determining whether fruit flies develop diet-related heart disease or not. Fruit flies on a time-restricted eating plan had hearts that seemed to be 20 to 30 per cent younger than their age would suggest. Furthermore, older fruit flies were able to develop healthier hearts when their time window for eating was reduced to 12 hours. Given that the hearts of fruit flies and human hearts are quite similar, it's quite possible that humans may similarly benefit from time-restricted eating in this way.

The science of intermittent fasting also highlights the benefits of enabling insulin levels to drop far enough and for long enough to enable you to burn more fat. Other potential benefits of time-restricted eating include reduced cellular inflammation and blood sugar, improved metabolism and brain functioning. Of course, if you have an underlying health condition, and particularly if you suffer from an eating disorder or are pregnant/breastfeeding, then time-restricted eating should only be considered under close medical supervision.

IN MY PRACTICE

I had another patient who struggled with this. Brian had been overweight ever since I had known him. A successful serial entrepreneur who travelled extensively for business across various time zones, he seemed to have time and energy for everything except his own health. To quote Brian, 'I felt fine and wasn't sick, so it just wasn't a priority for me.' While he did take some exercise, it was more sporadic than regular, and he often short-changed his sleep. His biggest blind spot was his eating habits, however. A diet heavy on the three Ss: salt, saturated fat and surplus calories (known by some as the SAD – Standard American Diet), and it was certainly light on nutrients and plant-based colour.

Having a heart attack at age 50 was a major wake-up call to Brian. He was luckier than most, getting to hospital quickly where a stent unblocked a critical artery in his heart. There was residual damage, but every chance he could make a good recovery. Provided, of course, that he changed his lifestyle habits.

Which is what I emphasised when I met up with Brian. Unlike his late father, who had died from a heart attack years earlier, Brian had been given a second chance. He had been lucky to survive and the next chapter was largely down to him. In essence, he had two questions to answer. Firstly, how important was good health to him? (Very, was his answer.) Secondly, how confident was he about making the changes? (Fairly, was his answer!)

My conversations with Brian enabled me to share two important ideas about eating habits. First was building the habit of mindful eating, developing awareness of his needs and being able to differentiate emotional and distracted eating from genuine hunger. Learning to score his hunger on a scale from one (ravenous) to ten (completely stuffed) supported Brian in building mindful awareness of his eating plan. Second was the importance of differentiating nutrients from calories in terms of a heart-healthy approach to his eating habits. He said that he found an episode of my podcast, In the Doctor's Chair, on the topic of the Mediterranean diet helpful to reinforce the basics. Brian did the rest. Today, almost a year later, Brian has transformed his attitude to food and nutrition.

He even grows his own vegetables. His belly has shrunk from 44 to 39 inches over that time. Great progress to date, and Brian has become a more mindful eater and a much more active participant in his own wellbeing.

THE MINDFUL EATING PRESCRIPTION

To bring the practice of more mindful eating into your life, I suggest you keep a written journal for a week or two (including weekends). Simply documenting what you're eating (in terms of the type and amount of food), the times you eat at and how you feel before and afterwards can give you fresh insights into your current eating patterns. This can deepen your conversation about more mindful eating and become a new starting point for more mindful change. I've put together a list of journal questions that will make a good starting point for your reflection.

Journal

o   When do I eat?

o   When do I shop, and where?

o   How do I feel when I'm shopping?

o   Do I have a list or do I shop on impulse?

o   What time do I have my first and last morsel of food or drink each day?

o   How often do I feel like eating or snacking?

o   Do I feel guilty when I eat?

o   Where do I eat?

o   Do I always eat seated at the kitchen table?

o   Do I buy snacks during my day?

o   Do I eat on the run?

o   What are my triggers for eating? Hunger or habit? Boredom, stress?

o   Do I crave food – and what types?

o   What times or situations bring on these cravings?

o   Are there times when I have willpower issues?

o   Are there any emotional triggers to eating, even though I'm not hungry?

o   Do I ever misunderstand hunger for feelings of stress, overwork or boredom?

o   Are there health issues that I'm aware of?

o   Have I tried diets?

o   How do I know when I'm hungry?

o   Do I drink enough water?

o   Have I tried quelling supposed hunger with water?

o   What do I eat on a typical day?

o   …on a night out?

o   …on a weekend?

o   What do I like to snack on?

o   What size plate do I use?

o   What's the one thing I could do to start eating more healthily?

o   What would success look like for me from an eating perspective?

o   How can I measure progress?

o   How can I reward myself for making this change?

o   What do I eat when I'm feeling stressed, bored, distracted?

o   Are there people, places or associations that trigger particular eating habits?

o   Do I eat quickly?

o   Do I savour my food?

o   How much do I eat?

o   Do I always clear my plate?

o   Do I tend to overeat?

o   How do I feel after I eat?

o   How do I use up the energy that food as fuel gives me – through exercise or movement?

The **Hunger Score** is a subjective scale to guide your own feelings when eating. It can be a helpful tool to build awareness about your eating habits, giving you insights to fine-tune your decision-making, and create a healthier and overall more satisfying relationship with food. The hunger scale enables you to better distinguish between emotional and physical hunger. This difference can be difficult to detect at first, given that the mind dictates what to eat and when.

Simply score yourself on the following scale before, during and after eating. The aim is to start eating when you score yourself a 3 or 4 on the scale, and to stop when you reach a 6. Consider it a rough guide – if the language used doesn't fit for you, then modify it into your own words. The idea is not about precision or perfection, simply to tune in to your body's feelings and need for food.

1. Ravenous: You are perhaps weak or even lightheaded. You will eat any food, even food you don't like.

2. Very hungry: Low energy, tummy growling.

3. Hungry: You have hunger pangs, and a strong desire to eat.

4. First signs of hunger: Awareness of wanting to eat.

5. Neutral: Comfortable. Neither hungry nor full.

6. Satisfied: No longer hungry. Satisfied, but could eat a few more bites.

7. Full: You are completely satisfied, perhaps even slightly uncomfortable. You have had enough, though your mind may tell you to have a little more.

8. Stuffed: You feel bloated and uncomfortable, overly full.

9. Very stuffed: Beyond stuffed. You feel way too full, uncomfortably so.

10. Overfull: The mere thought of more food might make you feel sick.

Practice makes improvement, so as you repeat this exercise, you become better self-attuned and feel more in control of your eating habits. It can support you to reduce eating for emotional reasons, comfort or boredom and more for genuine physical nourishment.

Before every meal:

O   Make sure you are well hydrated so you don't confuse hunger for thirst.

o   Bring your awareness to your stomach and score yourself
       on the hunger scale.

o   Typically, you will score about 3 if you are four hours or
       so since your last meal.

   During a meal

o   Stay attuned to your score as you eat mindfully. Pay
       attention for signals that you are no longer hungry and
       are comfortably satisfied.

o   Checking in half and three-quarters of the way through
       your meal can provide further insights into your degree
       of fullness. Try to stop when you reach 6 on the scale,
       even if your plate isn't empty.

   After a meal

o   Check in again with your score. Are you surprised with
       your score now?

Plan ahead: When you're hungry, you aren't always
thinking clearly; you're more likely to reach for the nearest
sweet or salty snack, whatever your stomach is growling for at
that time. Prepare for this by planning your snacks in advance
– have them within easy reach at home or in the office. You can
also consider your car as a health-enhancing environment,
and keep a water bottle and Tupperware box full of healthy
snacks stashed there.

A moment to pause: Before you start eating, take a
moment to appreciate and express gratitude for the food you
are about to eat, the people who prepared it, and those you

may be sharing the meal with. Make your meal a ritual, rather than something to be wolfed down on the run. Consider the cultural traditions involved or celebrated, the recipes, the ovens, saucepans and other equipment used. Extend your gratitude to the shops that supplied the food, the workers who stocked the shelves, the ingredients. Remember the natural elements in the creation of the food from the sun, soil, water, wind and rain. Those involved in the sowing, reaping and harvesting, the supply chains who supported them.

While you're eating, some further tips for remaining mindful include:

○   To slow yourself down, try using chopsticks or your non-dominant hand for utensils.

○   Chew slowly and attentively. Try to identify all the ingredients.

○   Take small bites and chew fully – up to 20–40 times with each mouthful.

○   Put utensils down in between bites.

More mindful eating is all about starting. Perhaps with one meal a day. It's all about progress. Taking a pause before you eat is a terrific technique for more progress towards mindful eating. Become aware of your real needs at that moment (which may be more for a kind word or comforting hug than a cookie). By building self-awareness, this enables you to tune in to your authentic self, and realign your choices with your real health goals.

SECTION THREE

The Soul of Vitality

The soul of vitality espouses connection through the inner journey to rediscover the essence of who you are, as well as a wider sense of connection in the world. This may include a spiritual act of faith, meditation or simple connection with nature. The aim is for you to find the courage to embrace your fears with a strong sense of self, bolstered by an understanding of *ikigai* (purpose) and meaning. Recharge and revitalise from life's stresses, while boosting your creativity. Experience simplicity and serenity with a deep sense of fulfilment and inner contentment.

Purpose:
finding yours

'A master in the art of living draws no sharp distinction between his work and his play; his labour and his leisure; his mind and his body; his education and his recreation. He hardly knows which is which.'

L.P. JACKS

Does this sound like you? Do you spend your day doing things you love to do? Doing things that matter, using your strengths? If so, you're one of the lucky ones, because lack of purpose has become a modern-day epidemic, with many people devoid of this spark and a real sense of who they are in the world. The result manifests in so many ways from addiction and accelerated burnout to adverse health conditions. In fact, more people suffer heart attacks early on Monday mornings than at any other time of the week, going to jobs they see as lacking purpose, meaning and fulfilment.

The United States agency Centers for Disease Control and Prevention has found that only one in every three people has a compelling reason to get up in the morning. So many people are searching for more meaning and purpose. More people than ever want to join the dots in their lives, to connect the personal and the professional, the scholarly and the spiritual. To reconnect what they do to who they are; to make a difference and meaningful contribution.

Modern life has a preoccupation with 'more' – more materialism, conspicuous consumption, endless comparison. While it's completely normal to want success and savour nice things in life, remember hedonic adaptation – the very real tendency to adapt to material comforts as they become part of the 'new normal'. It's little wonder how short-lived fulfilment from material things can be, unless or until a deeper sense of meaning and spiritual connection is found. Confucius, the Chinese philosopher, once wrote that you have two lives, with your second life starting the day you realise you only have one life. Living on purpose enables you to feel more alive, to be authentic and abundantly clear about those things that matter most.

So what is the true meaning of life? A great question, one of those timeless questions that has captivated scholars and sages throughout history. Here's the thing. No matter what your position or job title, irrespective of any professional qualifications you may hold, where you live or how many zeroes you have on your payslip, I believe the true meaning of life can be summed up in just one word: service.

THE BENEFITS OF PURPOSE

Imagine something so beneficial that it not only reduces risk of heart disease, stroke and dementia but dampens stress, builds resilience and enhances relationships. Increases your chances of staying alcohol and drug free after treatment. Puts more pep in your step (literally), potentially adding years to your life (and more life-filled vitality to your years). Helps you to stay more present throughout the day and even sleep better at night. Perhaps reduces your risk of early death even more than by exercising regularly – and that's saying a lot! Best of all, something that's freely available. 'Impossible,' I hear you say! But this substance does exist – it's called your purpose. Your unique ability to live a life of meaningful contribution, to make a difference, have an impact or master the art of fulfilment. Rediscovering the essence of your purpose is probably the most important determinant of your overall wellbeing.

Purpose supports healthier habits and behaviours, and builds more positive health-related choices. Of course, there may be an element of cause and effect here, as less healthy people may simply be less able to pursue hobbies or purposeful activities. Perhaps when you live with more purpose, you better value your own self-care and, as a consequence, take more proactive steps to mind your health.

While your work and career can provide tremendous meaning, retiring early can be associated with reduced longevity. Some people (men in particular) have a tendency to define themselves by what they do. The result, when they stop doing what they do, is the question: who are they? This is why retirement can be such a health hazard, especially for men, and why it is so important to redefine purpose in a much broader context. Having a direction in your life and developing overarching goals that transcend your job or how society can define you is so important, to protect you from major life transitions like retirement.

Purpose builds resilience. You are better able to handle the speedbumps of life and it provides an effective buffer against life's challenges. You build realistic optimism as you are better able to focus on what's most important – your 'north star' – your values and meaningful goals. This fuels focus, progress and more purpose in a synergistic upward spiral. Purpose can transform your view of stress, helping you to embrace it and enhance your potential to overcome setbacks, adversity and life's inevitable disappointments – leading to what is called post-traumatic growth. Purpose may be protective against the harmful effects of toxic stress, perhaps mediated through lower levels of stress hormones (cortisol levels) and lower blood pressure. Having more purpose in your life, whether that purpose comes from sea swimming, road running or volunteering for a cause you care about, provides a core psychological need to 'matter'.

Purpose is like glue in terms of how it strengthens authentic connection between mind, emotion, body and spirit. What you think, feel and do become more aligned with integrity of thought, word and deed. This creates a more seamless connection between head and heart, engaging you with the essence of who you are – raw, unscripted and real. You become more of a leader in your own life, empowered to own the choices you make with more clarity around what really matters. You are better able to accept yourself for who you really are – including your shortcomings and imperfections, as you embrace your challenges in life, on purpose. Living with purpose strengthens your sense of self and, by extension, your relationships with others, with higher levels of engagement seen between families, colleagues and community.

THE SCIENCE OF PURPOSE

Higher degrees of purpose may be protective against heart attack. Research at Mount Sinai Medical Center on more than 136,000 men and women has found that irrespective of how purpose is defined or the country involved, believing life is worth living with a sense of purpose and meaning leads to healthier hearts (lower cardiac events 19 per cent, mortality 23 per cent). Meanwhile, low levels of purpose were associated with increased risk of stroke, heart attack, stent or bypass surgery.

A large study, published in *The Lancet* in 2014, over eight years and involving 9,000 men aged over 65 years found that 29 per cent of those with the lowest purpose died (compared to nine per cent of those with the highest purpose). Those with highest purpose lived two years longer on average. A large study of 7,000 American adults aged 51 to 61, published in the *Journal of the American Medical Association*, found that those with a strong life purpose were less likely to die during the study period than those who didn't, and had a reduced risk of heart disease. This protective benefit of purpose may be more significant than not smoking, drinking to excess or even exercising regularly. Conversely, the association between having low levels of purpose and earlier death was independent of race, gender, wealth or education level.

The archipelago of Okinawa is home to some of the longest-living people in the world. It is a place where men and women tend to remain physically and mentally active, can be seen playing with their great, great, grandchildren, are connected to their gardens and to the world around them, often beyond the age of one hundred. Rates of chronic degenerative disease (from diabetes to dementia) are far less prevalent. There is no direct word for 'retirement' here, while the foundation stone to their philosophy of living is encapsulated by the word *ikigai* (pronounced eek-ee-guy). It is derived from:

○   -*iki*: meaning alive or life, and

○   -*kai*: meaning worth living, the realisation of dreams, hopes and expectations.

Ikigai translates as a reason for being, to include living with purpose, joy and a sense of wellbeing.

The concept of ikigai emerged from the timeless idea of interconnection with the elements of physical, mental and emotional health, all intertwining with one's purpose. Similar to the French phrase raison d'être, or reason for being, ikigai embellishes your entire life, enabling you to experience more positive emotions like joy, with a good reason to get up in the morning. Finding your ikigai, or letting it find you, is associated with greater feelings of happiness and fulfilment.

Ikigai is double-edged in that it includes both inner and outer purpose. Inner purpose is a sense of being (a feeling or spiritual meaning that life is worth living), while outer purpose is a sense of doing (the source of value in your life that is worth living for). In other words, having purpose for yourself while also providing benefit for others.

In the Ohsaki study of more than 40,000 Japanese men and women aged between 40 and 79, participants were asked a simple question: Do you have ikigai in your life?[33] Those without ikigai had increased mortality rates whereas in those who answered 'yes', more than 75 per cent had good or excellent self-rated health.

IN MY PRACTICE

This case study is slightly different from the others, in that this time, it's about my own journey. In Paulo Coelho's acclaimed book *The Alchemist* (one of my all-time favourites), the little shepherd boy Santiago was searching for the treasure in the Egyptian pyramids that he believed would bring him happiness. That story resonates with me because I, too, was searching for 'treasure' – in my case, career goals – only to become similarly disillusioned after I found it. While many of my professional goals were realised early on with 'success' as a medical doctor, I found myself caught up in becoming simply too busy. I allowed my self-awareness and inner voice to be drowned out by the relentless emotional demands of working as a GP at the coalface of primary healthcare.

Just after I had developed the Waterford Health Park in 2008, the world economy crashed. Closer to home, many people, particularly those in construction, lost their jobs, while many more had to deal with the double problem of next-to-no income on top of negative equity. There was a lot of fear and financial hardship, serious distress and, for many people I knew, a downward spiral into despair and depression. Tragically, lives were lost, families torn apart and futures fractured. Many young people without commitments emigrated, with many remaining trapped in a vicious spiral of debt demands.

During these times, I was luckier than most, with so much purposeful work to do in supporting others. Still, savage emergency financial cuts from the government made running a quality primary care service extremely difficult, especially in the face of relentless pressure from the bank. Keeping the show on the road as an employer wasn't easy for anyone in those dark days. While I had a great team of people around me, after a couple of years I began to feel worn out. Ironically, an unspoken 'truth' hardwired into medical training is that you are somehow supposed to be invincible, impervious to stress. Immune from the adverse effects of working around the clock, accepting sleep deprivation as something to admire and illness as something to admonish. Because fundamentally we, the doctors, were somehow different to 'them' – the patients.

My eventual experience of situational burnout was hardly a surprise in the circumstances. Caring is wearing. Ask many doctors about burnout and they may candidly say, 'Which burnout story do you want to hear?' Indeed, one in every three doctors may be experiencing burnout symptoms at any given time – just think about that the next time you pay your doctor a visit!

It's something I've seen many times over the years: people simply worn down, side-tracked or submerged in a tsunami of too much work. Combine this with a highly driven personality, inadequate 'switch-off' time and additional life stressors, including the deaths of a close family member and a lifelong friend, and you have the perfect recipe for situational burnout.

Learning to appreciate the importance of self-renewal and to invest more time in my own self-care enabled me to dampen down the noise, disconnect from the busyness of everyday life to reconnect with the essence of who I am. To rediscover and reconnect with my purpose, I asked myself four simple questions – which I'll return to later in the chapter – and spent time reflecting on and refining the answers.

Firstly, 'What am I good at?'

Secondly, 'What do I love to do?'

Thirdly, 'What does the world need?'

And finally, 'How can I be valued for my efforts?'

Doing this exercise confirmed my view that, for me, service *is* the meaning of life. Recommitting to use my strengths to serve others, while also taking good care of myself, is where the source of my joy and fulfilment really lies. And, in fact, my sense of purpose has been the silver lining in all of my professional challenges.

THE PURPOSE PRESCRIPTION

How do you live a more purposeful, authentic life, a life that allows you to be true to yourself and to your deepest values? Answering this question successfully goes a long way towards finding your ikigai and bringing more purpose into your everyday reality. Let me share some ideas that I have learned so far about authenticity, meaning and purpose. How, just like Santiago, you can rediscover what really matters to you and why.

Discovering your ikigai requires reflection and present-moment awareness. Asking the right questions opens the inner door to self-discovery, to define what real purpose means for you. In the words of the renowned psychiatrist and existential philosopher, Viktor Frankl, 'each man is questioned by life; and he can only answer to life by answering for his own life'.

Journal

Take quiet time to reflect on the questions below, which I believe will allow you to get in touch with the most real and authentic version of yourself and support you in creating a compelling purpose and narrative for your life.

O   How do you describe yourself in terms of the various roles in your life?

O   What do you want from life?

O   What do you really want?

O   What do you really, really want?

O   In other words, what matters most to you, as opposed to what's the matter!

O   How are you spending your time? Are your heart and mind telling you that you should be spending your time differently; doing different things?

O   Who are you becoming?

○ What do you want your life to stand for?

○ What makes your life worth living?

Positive health habits provide the energy and vitality to 'stay in contention', as I say. To make it possible to pursue your purpose or enable purpose to emerge from your everyday life. Let's take a look at the various areas of your life in which this should be addressed, and some ways in which you can do this.

Mind: Move from the outer world definition of what you have (based on possessions, pieces of paper or position in life) to who you are (determined by your values and sense of purpose which leads to real freedom). Present-moment awareness is the place where things unfold naturally with ease in alignment with your true nature and your purpose. Awareness can be cultivated through mindful meditation to various mindful practices (including mindful presence, mindful choice and mindful growth). When you move to 'being', through periods of stillness, silence or simply time immersed in nature, you become more reflective about the purpose and meaning of your life.

Emotion: Cultivating gratitude, realistic optimism, kindness and positive relationships builds a rich emotional bank account of positivity which underpins purpose. In turn, purpose can generate a ripple effect of positive contagion throughout your life, nurturing curiosity and creativity.

Physical: Invest enough time and energy into the foundations of great physical health – including restorative sleep, mindful eating and regular movement. Better awareness and more insightful choices will help you become more closely aligned to your life's purpose.

Spiritual: The word 'spirituality' comes from the Latin word *spiritus* (meaning soul, courage, breath). Spiritual wellbeing cultivates gratitude and positive emotions including hope and inspiration. It builds resilience, inner peace and serenity. You become more 'other-centred' in terms of compassion and concern, while also deepening your own sense of purpose and meaning.

I call spiritual health 'soulful connectivity'. It is the essence of your being; your inner life and its relationship with your outer life. As a subjective search for the sacred, this relationship with your higher power includes concepts such as inner peace, purpose and prayer. Spirituality forms the backbone of those guiding principles that support and motivate you as you move through life, like a compass giving your life its overall direction. Spiritual health is defined by your values, beliefs, morals, principles and faith. Some questions you can ask when looking to delve deeper into your spiritual health include:

o   Do you make time for prayer, meditation or reflection on the meaning of life events?

o   Do you make time for silence?

o   Do you find it easy to forgive others ... and to forgive yourself?

o   Are you compassionate?

o   Are your choices and decisions guided by your values?

o   Are you tolerant and considerate of the views of others, which may well be different from your own?

If you answered 'No' to any of these questions, it may provide an opportunity to enhance your spiritual health and wellbeing. This can be an intensely personal experience, involving beliefs and values that provide purpose and meaning for you in your own life. What works best for you may not work as well for someone else. Be willing to experiment a little and see what fits you best. Here are some ways – both large and easily achievable – in which you can look to improve your spiritual wellbeing.

Find your team: Invest in your relationships and connect with people that share your values and make you feel recognised, valued and appreciated. Because of the power of social contagion, your associations can have a big impact on your outlook, action and capacity to live your purpose.

Value your values: Live your own values, while trying to make a more positive difference in the world. Values are freely chosen, providing freedom from comparison and strengthening your sense of self, particularly self-acceptance. Hold yourself to the standards you believe in as an active, living demonstration of your values. Actions do speak louder than words.

Volunteer: Consider volunteering for a cause you believe in. Give more of your time, talents and energy to serve others more, build a better world and make a contribution based on your own unique strengths and interests. Instead of looking at what's in it for you, you are outwardly asking how you can better support others. To make more of a difference, to be the difference.

Micro-moments of purpose: Write down a few moments in your week that stand out in terms of purpose and meaning. It may be something very small, sharing a coffee and conversation with a friend, seeing a beautiful sunset.

Micro-environments of purpose: Create visual reminders in your work and home of those things that matter most to you. Put a meaningful photo, image or quote on the wallpaper of your phone and computer as a regular reminder.

Craft your life: Life crafting is an exercise that focuses on positive psychology principles that support health and vitality (known as salutogenesis). Schippers and Ziegler of Erasmus University formally defined life crafting as 'a process in which people actively reflect on their present and future life, set goals for important areas of life – social, career and leisure time – and, if required, make concrete plans and undertake actions to change these areas in a way that is more congruent with their values and wishes'. By actively reflecting on your present and future life, goals consistent with your values in important areas (professional, personal, pastimes, etc.) along with publicly expressed plans to make positive changes and actions in alignment with what matters most to you. It includes writing answers to questions on the following:

Journal

O   What are you passionate about (your interests)?

O   What do you value (what's important to you)?

O   What goals in your life are consistent with your own values, rather than the expectations of others? Setting and working towards goals that are self-determined and self-motivated can be an important element of your wellbeing and vitality.

○ What's your current VitalityMark? What's your intention gap between your current and future VitalityMark?

○ What are your plans to achieve these goals and how might you navigate the inevitable speed bumps (or roadblocks!) that arise along the way?

○ How would you describe your best possible future self? How might it feel when everything you work towards comes to pass? Another important element to the life crafting exercise is to commit publicly to the goals you set, moving you from 'I'd like to ...' to 'I will ...'

Writing about your goals can build resilience to setbacks and increase the likelihood of them coming to pass. They satisfy basic psychological needs of competence, autonomy and relatedness. As such, they build a sense of purpose and meaning.

Answering the question of what your ikigai is may not come naturally to you, or indeed to many people. Not to worry, there's help on hand. Answering these four questions will make it easier for you and likely to provide some clues to your ikigai.

Firstly, what do you love to do? In other words, what brings you joy and fulfilment? What makes you feel energised and engaged, most alive? What activities cause you to lose track of time? What might you continue to do, even for free? When do you feel happiest? How can you do more of what you love to do? Are you willing to follow your heart, find your flow, do what you love *and* learn to love what you do?

Secondly, what are you good at? What are your strengths, skills and talents? What do you excel at? What comes naturally to you? What are your hobbies? What do people ask you for advice or support with? What's your 'unique selling point'?

Thirdly, what does the world need? In terms of 'the world' this can be either a global issue affecting the entire planet or something local to your own community or neighbourhood. How can you contribute more? Where can you make a difference? What challenges would you like to help solve? How can you better support others?

Fourthly, how are you valued? This might be your job or career, in terms of what you can be paid for, or else it could simply be the fulfilment derived from volunteering. If you weren't in your current job, what might you do? Could you make a living doing this in the longer term? If so, what fears are holding you back? In other words, what's stopping you from starting?

The four circles in the diagram on the next page may be a more Westernised version of ikigai. The pure Japanese version is simply doing what you love, in alignment with the Zen principles of simple being. Having a sense of mindful presence, discovering joy in little everyday things and finding flow in one's lived experience. From this version, you can see that:

O   At the intersection of what you love and what you are good at is your **Passion**.

○ At the intersection of what you love and what the world needs is your **Mission**.

○ At the intersection of what you are good at and what you can get paid for is your **Profession**.

○ At the intersection of what the world needs and what you can get paid for is your **Vocation**.

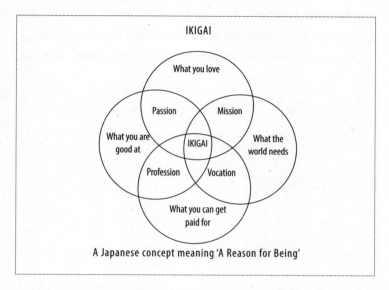

IKIGAI

What you love

Passion

Mission

What you are good at

IKIGAI

What the world needs

Profession

Vocation

What you can get paid for

A Japanese concept meaning 'A Reason for Being'

Purpose as a word is often misrepresented as some cause celebre or special kind of mission to save the world. *Real* purpose is understanding that you don't need to change the world, because chances are, you can't. But with courage and conviction, you can choose to change yourself. Purpose is something that ensues from exploring the essence of who you are. As an inside job, purpose comes from your values, your strengths, from what makes your heart sing. Your purpose is always there, waiting for you to rediscover it.

More than anything, you build purpose into your life. You build it from your past, your experiences, values, talents and abilities. You build it from your family and community, from the people and causes you care about. These are the raw ingredients of purpose. Only you can reconfigure them together in an authentic manner that is your life.

Perhaps the real rewards for embracing purpose and inspiration were espoused more than two thousand years ago by the poetic words of that great teacher from India, Patañjali:

> When you are inspired by some great purpose, some extraordinary project, all your thoughts break their bonds; your mind transcends limitations, your consciousness expands in every direction and you find yourself in a new, great and wonderful world. Dormant forces, faculties and talents become alive, and you discover yourself to be a greater person by far than you ever dreamed yourself to be.

Day by day, you can adjust your mindset and perspective from 'what you can take from life today' to 'how you can contribute to life today'. In this way, the essence of purpose – your ikigai – becomes a catalyst for a life of more vitality.

Meditation:
an inner key

'You shouldn't chase after the past or place expectations on the future.
What is past is left behind. The future is yet unreached. Whatever
quality is present you clearly see right there, right there.'

BUDDHA

As a spiritual practice, meditation is seen in Sanskrit Indian philosophy and structured religion from Christianity to Buddhism. In recent times, it has been 'rediscovered' as a key experiential tool for more mindful living. For me, this is perhaps the greatest opportunity that meditation provides: more presence and attentive awareness as a key part of everyday experience.

Many people who suffer from toxic stress can benefit from a mindful practice like meditation. While it's something I often recommend, there can be pushback to this suggestion. Many people believe that meditation is not for them, that they are not that 'type of person'. Some say they are simply too busy to add yet another item onto their 'to do' list. Some stop because they don't experience any 'buzz' or immediate positive change. Others comment how they can't stop their 'merry-go-mind' of anxious negative thoughts from racing.

Do you agree with any or some of the following statements?

○   I feel stressed.

○   I feel anxious.

○   I have a diminished sense of self.

○   I feel pessimistic.

○   I feel stuck in a rut.

○   I find it hard to concentrate.

○   My energy and vitality are low.

○   I feel unenthusiastic and uninspired.

○   I feel flat.

○   My relationships are a source of stress.

○   I am worrying a lot.

○   I am easily distracted.

○   I am poor at handling conflict.

○   My mind is always racing.

If so, then you're not alone – far from it. As I mentioned earlier, your 'merry-go-mind' of anxious negative thoughts can unleash an inner critic that plays havoc with your wellbeing. While you have many, many thoughts each day, you are not your thoughts. As an analogy, consider your mobile phone. While it receives text messages (thoughts), your phone is much more than any or all of the messages it receives. Similarly, you have thoughts, but you are not your thoughts. While you may have upwards of 6,000 thoughts a day (most of them negative), it is those thoughts you pay attention to that have a major impact on who you are and become. Thoughts you hold on to can trigger beliefs, feelings and behaviours that are emotionally exhausting. Thoughts you hold on to can tell you stories about your life and how the world works that simply aren't true. This can create a mindset of scarcity and mediocrity and a rigidity to your thinking in terms of how you see things. In short, living in the clutches of your untamed ego, driven by fear and scarcity, what I call chronic not-enoughness.

Nowadays, with the never-ending news cycle of crisis and conflict in a world of constant competition and comparison, people have never been more prone to distress and distraction. Add in the turmoil of addiction, anxiety and isolation and it's easy to understand why a tsunami of toxic stress and burnout is taking a major toll on the health and vitality of individuals everywhere. Healthcare is no exception either. Caring can be, and often is so, wearing. All of these factors create an unarguable case for meditation. To rebalance your inner world of thought and emotion with your outer lived experience. To slow down, press pause and create a more mindful awareness of your natural state of being.

Some people embrace meditation when suffering from stress, then desist once the source of their stress has abated – seeing the practice as more of a short-term fix than a longer-term way of life. This is perfectly understandable, but unfortunate, given that meditation is so much more than a band-aid for a bad day. What's clear is that meditation can enhance so many aspects of your wellbeing, supporting greater levels of life success, whether you define this by your resilience and relationships, accomplishments, achievements and self-leadership, or simply allowing yourself to be more still and present.

Admittedly, meditation takes time, an investment of as little as five to ten minutes a day. Moreover, it is a commitment to press the pause button on your life, to journey inwards to that place of inner stillness. Traditionally, meditation was considered in the West to be something that you either believed in or (more often) didn't. Indeed, I myself used to believe that meditation was for people who lived on the other side of the world, probably reclusive monks who had nothing better to do all day than sit around and meditate. Light years away from my life and work as a busy family doctor. Even when I read some research about the documented brain changes on FMRI scans in long-term meditators (more than 10,000 hours each) my reaction – like many, not unreasonably – was 'Sure, I don't have 10,000 hours available.' Not many people do, as 10,000 hours equates to nearly two and a half hours a day, each and every day for 10 years! More recently, research has emerged to suggest that that as little as 11 hours of cumulative meditative practice (not all together!) can lead to brain changes, including calming the stress centre (amygdalae) and boosting self-awareness[34]. This works out at about 10 minutes a day for three months, and, given the potential benefits, now I was interested enough to take action.

That was several years ago. Building a meditation habit, just like any new habit, takes time and that's okay. Nothing worthwhile is easy. The key is consistency, to never stop starting.

THE SCIENCE OF MEDITATION

While the precise mechanisms by which meditation 'works' remain unclear, the mechanics of the human brain are under active investigation. One of the key ideas to emerge thus far from this fascinating field of neuroscience is what's known as the Hebbian Principle. This means that your brain can be stretched, strengthened and developed over time, just like a muscle.

Far from being hardwired, your brain is live-wired from your everyday experiences in life. This occurs through a process known as neuroplasticity, whereby the brain can change and evolve right throughout your lifetime (and not just when you are a child or teenager). Cells that fire together, wire together.

Richard Davidson, from the University of Wisconsin, has been one of the first scientists to suggest that meditation can alter brain structure. As I mentioned previously, FMRI scans on Tibetan monks who were experienced meditators (meditating on cultivation of compassion through loving-kindness) were found to experience a massive increase in gamma brainwave activity. This was seen particularly in the left prefrontal cortex, a brain area which is the seat of positive emotions like enthusiasm, happiness and joy (as opposed to the right prefrontal cortex which is associated with negative emotional states like sadness and anxiety). In other words, meditation can influence the structure of your brain, making it more receptive to positivity, as the happiness centre in the brain becomes bigger.

The type of brainwaves emitted from the brain during meditation can be seen to change from predominantly beta waves, associated with the busyness of the 'merry-go-mind', to more alpha wave activity, associated with deep relaxation.

The frequency of brainwaves is correlated with differing mental states.

○   **Delta waves:** seen in deep sleep. 0.1–4 Hz

○   **Theta waves:** seen in trance states and the preconscious state just before falling asleep and waking up. 4–8Hz

○   **Alpha waves:** seen in a relaxed but alert state of consciousness seen; best when eyes are closed. 8–13Hz

○   **Beta waves:** most of the brain is in this state when your eyes are open and you are making decisions and processing the world around you. May relate to the anxious alertness of the 'merry-go-mind'. 13Hz +

○   **Gamma waves:** seem to indicate interconnection between vast areas of brain tissue. Turning separate elements of data into a single experience. They may be related to the loss of self and sense of interconnection experienced in deep meditative states. They are needed for higher levels of mental activity, including self-awareness, perception, fresh insights and information processing. 30Hz +

Neuroplastic brain changes with meditation have been especially noted in the hippocampus (associated with learning and memory) as well as brain areas associated with awareness, cognitive focus, compassion and reflection.

Research from Massachusetts General Hospital and Harvard Medical School has shown that meditation increases the density of grey matter in areas of the brain associated with self-awareness, stress regulation, memory, empathy, and learning[35]. Several areas of the brain tend to become more active during meditation. A meta-analysis of 21 studies, which examined the brains of 300 seasoned meditators, found that several different brain areas were consistently changed as a result of meditation[36]: changes in brain thickness and density, white matter fibre density, cortical surface area as well as an increase in the numbers of brain cells (neurons) in a given area.

While research into the specific potential benefits of meditation is ongoing, it appears that it may impact many different brain regions simultaneously with compound benefits accumulating over time. Fascinating research from the Max Planck Society and published in *Science Advances* also suggests that different types of meditation can impact the brain differently. In the study, carried out on people aged 20 to 50 years of age, each participant underwent three separate types of meditation training for three months in duration. Brain scans were carried out at the start of the research and again at three-monthly intervals. Results showed that different meditation techniques can bring about nuanced brain changes.

In the first module, called **Presence**, the meditation was about focused attentive awareness, on the breath and internal bodily sensations. This Presence meditation led to brain scan changes of thickening in the anterior cingulate gyrus and prefrontal cortex and those brain areas strongly associated with attention. The second module was called **Affect**, which was a loving-kindness (also known as Metta) meditation training designed to enhance empathy and compassion. As predicted, this was associated with brain thickenings in areas of the brain dealing with social emotions such as empathy. The third module, **Perspective**, was very similar to mindful meditation. It focused on open observation of one's thoughts without judgement, while increasing understanding of the perspectives of others. This was associated with brain thickenings in areas corresponding to inhibiting the perspective of self while increasing understanding of others.

THE BENEFITS OF MEDITATION

Meditation aims to build self-awareness while enhancing emotional and attentional self-regulation – all key capacities of the self. The benefits appear to be cumulative, just like compound interest. Quite simply, the more you meditate, the better the results. Little wonder it is increasingly recognised as a key practice for successful leadership.

One of the most reported benefits of mindful meditation is a **buffer against stress**. While the brain can manage moderate amounts of stress, chronic or prolonged stress (without sufficient recharge) exposes the brain to damage. Areas dealing with self-regulation and fear-based memories appear most susceptible, including the amygdalae, prefrontal cortex and hippocampus. Chronic stress appears to increase the size of the amygdalae and reduce the size of the prefrontal cortex. The good news is these changes from chronic stress are considered malleable, and open to change with positive inputs from a mindful meditative practice. Mindful meditation is thought to alleviate stress by one of two ways. Firstly, it increases vagal tone, enhancing the parasympathetic nervous system, thereby reducing the sympathetic (fight or flight) response. Secondly, mindful meditation enhances self-regulation and self-control through neuroplasticity changes in the prefrontal cortex and hippocampus with a reduction in the amygdalae. Overall, mindful meditation can become a wonderful pathway towards a healthier, more resilient mind, thereby boosting overall vitality.

Meditation can be a wonderful way into **self-awareness**; to declutter your brain from the distractions of the 'merry-go-mind' and disconnect from the certainty of 'knowing', judging, labelling or comparing. To detach from thought itself, and to simply be. Imagine the ripple effect in a very still pond after you throw in a pebble. This is how your enhanced level of awareness can detect even the slightest ripple from the stillness. Without quietening your mind through meditation, a tidal wave could crash through your mind and you might not blink an eye or even notice a thing. In a world of socially prescribed perfectionism, meditation cultivates a mind that is willing to embrace uncertainty, open to everything and attached to 'no-thing'. To see things more openly – just like a child – or with what Zen masters call the 'beginner's mind'. Where you place your attention and awareness matters. While you can pay attention to many different things, when your attentive awareness pays attention to attention itself, then the stillness that ensues can open the door to your inner self. This is an opportunity to explore your own sense of self, in terms of 'who am I?' As you go deeper and deeper into meditation, detaching from your 'merry-go-mind' dissolves emotions and memories away as your self-identity disappears. Eventually all that remains is empty space, ever expanding, effortless and boundless. As you lose your sense of time, you rest in stillness; a beautiful, restful place where there is no noise, no ego, no memory, thought or time, no-thing except *you*.

Mindful meditation may help to build a more **resilient brain**, through neuroplasticity changes in areas of the brain involved in attention control and emotional regulation. With the former, brain regions important for attention control show structural and functional changes following the practice of mindfulness meditation. Cognitive control in the prefrontal cortex is enhanced while activity in the amygdalae is reduced. Enhanced levels of emotional regulation are also seen with mindfulness meditation. This includes how emotions emerge (in what situation, how long they last), how they are experienced and expressed. Overall, the intensity and frequency of negative effect tends to be reduced while positive mood states are improved.

Meditation strengthens your willpower muscle, making it easier to build and maintain new habits, successfully break old habits or set and work towards goals consistent with your values. It supports grit, graft and builds resilience. You become more willing to accept and take responsibility for things as they really are, as opposed to how you think they should, could or must be.

Success can be a difficult word to define. Traditionally, it is associated with external measures – achievement, attainment, accomplishments – and the idea of the destination, that 'I'll be successful when ... I have a bigger job, or car or house'. I like to define success differently, as an inside-out job that can start this very moment. Inner fulfilment is the starting point for true success, appreciating that right here, this very moment, 'I am enough, I have enough.' As the saying goes, the person who has enough is the person who knows they have more than enough! As an aside, many CEOs of the world's leading companies now include a meditative practice as part of their self-care strategy. Furthermore, meditation can enhance your degree of life success if you can define success by any or all of the following criteria:

Cultivation of compassion: Loving-kindness meditation is thought to boost compassion by dampening activity in the amygdalae in the presence of suffering, while activating brain circuits that build feelings of love and positivity. As a result, it can prompt you to take action to alleviate someone's suffering. As a mindful practice, it seems to activate part of the brain involved in empathy and emotional regulation (the left anterior insula/inferior frontal gyrus). By plugging you into the vagus nerve, the release of oxytocin hormone enhances empathy and builds connection.

Vitality of mind: The brain is known to be a very energy-intense organ, consuming at least 20 per cent of the body's energy even though it only accounts for two per cent of the body's size. Mindful presence through meditation minimises the diffusion of blood flow through the brain (this happens when you are stressed or distracted), supporting more efficient use of brain energy. Eight weeks of mindfulness-based stress reduction (MBSR) has been shown to reduce symptoms of depression and anxiety while enhancing wellbeing. Mindfulness meditation builds self-awareness as you move away from a static concept of self towards a more fluid dynamic sense of experiencing and being. This leads to a more positive self-image, higher levels of self-confidence and self-esteem. Meditation supports a stronger sense of self, as you become more aware, attuned and attentive to your thoughts, emotions and interactions with others. As you clear away the 'brain fog' and deepen mental clarity, you become more confident, more open to new ideas and imaginative insights. As a result, your sense of creativity and innovation is enhanced. As you develop mastery over your attentive awareness, you will be less prone to distraction, both from your external environment and from the internal environment of the 'merry-go-mind'. You become better able to be less reactive and more responsive, better able to reflect on experiences and situations.

Physical vitality: Benefits on physical health and vitality are particularly important in the Western world where the emphasis is on science. By contrast, meditation in the East is seen as a path to wisdom, higher states of consciousness and enlightenment. Physically, meditation can support a stronger immune system, making you better able to fight infections. It can reduce your perception of chronic pain and support better biological ageing. Physically, meditators tend to have enhanced levels of telomerase, an enzyme that slows biological ageing and supports cell regeneration, telomere function and longevity. Whether this is caused solely by meditation or other factors has yet to be determined.

Heart health: What's good for the head often tends to be good for the heart! The habit of regular meditation may play a beneficial role in reducing your risk of heart disease. According to the *Journal of the American Heart Association*, a review of numerous studies published over the past two decades has found that meditation can support heart health by improving many factors linked with heart disease, including helping to lower raised blood pressure. An American Heart Association scientific statement published in *Hypertension* (and which pooled data from nine separate studies) found that meditation made a modest but measurable difference to blood pressure. On average, meditation was found to lower systolic blood pressure (the top number in a blood pressure reading) by 4.7 milligrams of mercury (mm Hg) and diastolic blood pressure (the bottom number in the blood pressure reading) by 3.2 mm Hg.

Heart Rate Variability (HRV) is a measure of heart health that reflects how rapidly your heart makes small changes in the time interval between each heartbeat. (Normally, your heart rate speeds up slightly as you breathe in and slows slightly as you breathe out. The variance between these two rates is the

HRV.) A higher HRV is a sign of a healthier heart while a lower HRV has been found to be associated with an increased risk of heart attack or stroke among people without cardiovascular disease. Regular meditation (perhaps as little as five minutes of meditation daily for 10 days) can boost HRV.

Emotional vitality: Meditation can boost your emotional agility, empathy and compassion while enhancing emotional fulfilment. It builds your emotional bank account with more positivity, supporting inner happiness and wellbeing. It enhances your capacity to flow with, rather than fight against, your emotions. To name and tame, embrace and erase emotion in a manner that allows you to work with rather than work against them. As you clear your mind of destructive, toxic emotions, you become calmer and more at ease as you contribute to your own sense of inner peace and serene contentment.

Spiritual vitality: *Samadhi* is a Sanskrit term for a state of intense meditative concentration, whereby through the practice of meditation you experience higher consciousness, unity and a sense of oneness with the universe. Meditation enables you to engage more completely with the essence of who you are. Fostering a natural state of stillness, restful presence and inner peace. As your perspective changes, meditation can align you more closely to your values and sense of purpose, supporting your growth in awareness, inner 'knowing' and intuitive wisdom.

Connection: Meditation promotes balance and supports connections between emotion, body, mind and spirit. It strengthens relationships with others, building inner fulfilment and happiness. Furthermore, meditation can be a catalyst for robust relationships with positive associations between the quality of a relationship and mindfulness.

IN MY PRACTICE

One of the privileges of working as a family doctor is that you can become an astute observer of human experience. Not just what someone says, but how they are while they say it. Which reminds me of Stephen, probably the most Zen-like Irish person I have ever met. As someone who exudes inner calm and presence, it was little surprise for me to learn that Stephen had been meditating regularly for many years. In his former career in financial services, he had 'worn the golden handcuffs' – Stephen's description of how he had felt trapped by the never-ending relentless grind in his work as a corporate financier. The day he deplaned a transatlantic flight to find there were more than two hundred emails in his inbox became his tipping point to a career change. A chance meeting with a spiritual monk led him to a meditation retreat, and, as he says, the rest is history. 'I was initially attracted to meditation, thinking it would reduce my stress levels, which it did. However, I have stayed with the practice for the lasting benefits from regularly gifting my mind periods of stillness.' He describes the feelings of inner calm and serenity he can experience from simply being fully engaged in present-moment awareness. He says he gets far less bothered by life's mini hassles and feels far more in control of his life overall.

Now, years later, as a teacher of meditation, Stephen shares his experience and insights with others, running regular restorative retreats while continuing to further deepen his 'discovery of the beginner's mind, open to everything while attached to no-thing'.

THE MEDITATION PRESCRIPTION

Choose a space that is quiet and free from distractions. If you must have your phone close by, put it on silent mode. Find a comfortable posture. My personal preference is to sit still, in a relaxed position, on a chair with my legs uncrossed and feet flat on the ground. I've learned from experience that lying down may cause you to fall asleep! A good supportive posture is important, as it gives more freedom to the passage of air as you breathe.

Place your hands on your thighs with your palms facing upwards. Close your eyes and position your tongue onto the roof of your mouth behind your front two teeth. Scan your body and relax any tension. Let your spine rise from the ground of the pelvis. Draw your chin slightly down and let the back of your neck lengthen as you simply concentrate all your attention on your breath. Breathe slowly and steadily, over and over again. As you inhale through your nose, air flows in turn through your nostrils towards your throat, bronchial tubes and finally to the bottom of your lungs before reversing its direction as you breathe out through your nose again.

Your breath is an essential bodily rhythm that is connected to blood pressure, heart rate, mood and stress response. The breathing centre is close to the stress centre in the brain and, as you slow your breathing with attention and awareness, you dampen feelings of stress while building feelings of calm and relaxation. Learn to allow your breathing to be led by your attention and to let your attention rest on your breath. Please be patient. No self-judgement on your efforts, or expectations for a certain outcome. Let the effort of simply engaging with the practice of meditation become its own reward.

It can take a lot of practice and effort to keep your mind still, free from the 'merry-go-mind' of all those anxious negative thoughts. Some might say it can take a lifetime! In fact, it is inevitable that your mind will wander to the outside world, with concerns of the past or worries about the future. That's absolutely okay; it happens even to the most experienced meditators. Simply bring your awareness back to your breath if and (more likely when) your mind wanders. The key is to accept this, to not judge your judgements, and start again. Commit to the journey of meditation, and never stop starting.

There are two main types of meditation. Firstly, traditional mindful meditation, which is all about decluttering the 'merry-go-mind' through non-judgemental attention to present-moment experience. Secondly, loving-kindness meditation, as espoused by the Dalai Lama, which emphasises the radiation of compassion and love outwards from your heart. This can be a powerful antidote to feelings of hostility, anger or other toxic emotions.

Beyond these, other popular meditation practices include:

Mantra meditation: This is similar to the mindful breath meditation above, except your focus here is on a specific mantra as you breathe in and out. The mantra 'So Hum' is often used in this way for its vibrational impact rather than any specific meaning per se. Many people describe a deeper more meaningful experience when meditating with a mantra. Simply use the word 'So' each time as you inhale and 'Hum' as you exhale. Reflect on the word slowly and quietly as you breathe. An alternative is to simply think of the term 'So Hum' and let it go as you continue to breathe slowly and steadily. Repeat the mantra regularly as it arises in your mind.

Pranayama: This is an ancient breathing technique from the yoga tradition that focuses on the breath. Here, you alternate breaths through your left and right nostrils. It's much easier than it sounds! Sit upright and place your left hand over your nose such that your thumb is over your left nostril and the two middle fingers are against the right nostril. Gently close the right nostril and inhale through the left. Then exhale through the left nostril, move your thumb to close that nostril and release your fingers to open your right nostril. Now breathe in and out through your right nostril, before repeating the process. Every second breath is through the left or right nostrils. Breathe naturally and steadily in this manner for five minutes before doing your guided meditation in the usual manner. While it can take more effort than simple meditation, people who make Pranayama a habit often report a deeper meditative experience. Try it and see for yourself.

Informal meditation: There are many informal types of meditation you can engage in regularly. Spend time silently communing with nature, watching the sun rise, listening to the sound of birds chirping or water flowing in a stream.

Derived from the Sanskrit root *yuj*, which means 'to unite', yoga promotes unity of mind, body and spirit. Yoga teaches balance, between mind and body, mind and spirit. Other mindful body exercises such as tai chi or Pilates also emphasise mental focus, slow intentional movements and focused breathing. These are all a type of informal meditation, as are other varieties of steady repetitive rhythmic movements such as swimming or simply walking in nature.

Whatever method you opt for, whether it's sitting with your eyes closed and paying attention to your breathing, or simply immersing yourself in stillness through nature, the practice of mindful meditation illuminates awareness of your inner self, with numerous potential benefits. There is no consensus or fixed answer to the question of how much meditation is optimal or how often. I believe a little is better than none, and more is better than a little. To quote St Francis de Sales, 'I meditate for half an hour each day unless I'm busy, then I meditate for a full hour.' Ultimately, you will decide what is best for you.

Viriditas:
revitalising nature

'The effect of nature's qualities on health are not only spiritual and emotional but physical and neurological. I have no doubt that they reflect deep changes in the brain's physiology, and perhaps even its structure.'

OLIVER SACKS

Time for another imagination workout. This time, imagine a prescription that you can take and repeat indefinitely, replenishing your mental and physical health, restoring emotional energy and overall vitality. A prescription with no known side effects, it's also completely free. A gateway from doing to being, enabling you to feel refreshed and recharged, at ease with a sense of serenity and inner peace. Sounds, sights, scents and smells that soak up your stress and plug you into a bigger connection with the universe. For me that place is nature, especially among trees. Being in nature can feel so comforting, restorative and rejuvenating. The sounds of birds singing, seeing the speckled sunlight through the leaves, the scents and aromas, the atunement of the senses. Welcome to the concept of a green exercise prescription – spending time outdoors in nature for health and vitality.

For years, I have had an intuitive sense that being in nature is a health-enhancing environment, informed not just by my own experiences but by those of so many others. Spending time in nature can be simply so restorative and relaxing, a tremendous way to destress after a busy day at work. Moreover, I have found the beautiful Mount Congreve gardens close to where I live to be my 'creative laboratory', providing mental clarity and a sense of peaceful equanimity. Many of my patients have benefitted as well, which led me to begin prescribing a 'walk in nature' as a therapeutic tool back in 2017 in collaboration with Mount Congreve.

Significant research from the University of Exeter involving more than 20,000 people and published in the journal *Scientific Reports* in 2019 has found that people who spend at least 120 minutes a week in nature (whether at the one time or cumulatively throughout the week) are far more likely to report better physical health and psychological wellbeing than those who either didn't spend time in nature at all, or whose total time per week was less than 120 minutes. This time threshold of 120 minutes held for people of all age groups, from diverse backgrounds and social standings. Irrespective of how close someone lived to green spaces or how often someone spent time there, significant benefits accrued from a total exposure of 120 minutes over the entire week. Spending longer may provide additional benefits, though further research is needed to determine this. This scientific backing for my intuitive sense has led me on a journey of discovery, to dig deeper and delve into the health-boosting vitality of nature.

Viriditas is a term for the vitality-enhancing life force which emanates from nature, first described by Hildegard of Bingen – a twelfth-century philosopher nun, poet and polymath. Originating from the Latin words for green (*viridis*) and truth (*veritas*), viriditas symbolises the breadth and beauty of creation, from the vitality of the human spirit to the healing benefits of nature. Not just in terms of the potential of plants to produce fruits and fragrance, but the potential of humans to grow and flourish. By contrast, its opposite was described as ariditas – the dry and diminished sense of physical and spiritual vitality that results from not cultivating viriditas in your life. Caring for your physical environment enhances your sense of autonomy and builds connection to the world around you. This supports an expanded sense of self-care – including care for your environment and the world you live in. By placing nature and greenness at the very centre, viriditas highlights the interconnection between the vitality of the individual and the vitality of the planet. That people exist as the microcosm within the macrocosm of the universe. A powerful reminder that cultivating viriditas in your everyday habits leads to more vitality in mind, body and soul.

Biophilia is the scientific term for the biological need to connect with nature. The term originates from Greek, meaning 'love of life and the living world'. This concept was popularised by American biologist E.O. Wilson, who said, 'Our existence depends on this propensity, our spirit is woven from it, hope rises on its currents.' While no specific genes have been identified as of yet, there is a growing awareness of how the environments you spend your time in impact your epigenome. Biophilia explains the desire for the view of nature or the sea so sought after by many home dwellers. Spending time in nature is 'hardwired' into your physiology and enhances health in its broadest sense of mind, body, emotion and spirit. Nature can bridge the gap between doing and being and is a key driver of vitality and viriditas.

Do you spend much of your time indoors? Or do you take time to regularly immerse yourself in nature? Unfortunately, if you have the lifestyle habits of a typical person, you spend at least 90 per cent of your time indoors, with much of that 'indoor-itis' spent on digital devices – more than eight hours a day on average. I call this **nature deficit disorder**, where you lose out on the restorative benefits of time in nature, not just in terms of how you feel, but for recharge from stress and longer-term epigenetic expression.

THE SCIENCE OF NATURE

When Isaac Newton pondered the concept of gravity – 'what goes up must come down' – his eureka moment supposedly happened when an apple hit him on the head as he sat under a tree. No coincidence that he was out in nature at the time, subconsciously soaking up all the mental clarity and creativity-boosting benefits of a natural environment. Time outdoors in nature enables the prefrontal cortex to unplug for a while. This is the logical, rational part of the brain in charge and control of executive planning, preparation, decision-making, inhibition and social expression. This 'brain break' can result in a change in the quality of your thinking, reducing stress while enhancing creativity.

The amygdalae are the almond-shaped set of neurons that play a key role in the processing of emotions, including fear and anxiety. Spending time in nature quietens the amygdalae, moving you away from the fight or flight, always-on, highly wired state of your (beta wave) busy mind, towards a more pause and plan, chilled out (alpha wave) relaxed state. Alpha waves boost mood through the release of serotonin. Factor in lower levels of stress hormones and inflammatory marker IgA, and nature becomes a terrific way to reduce ruminations and feelings of anxiety. Spending time in nature builds resilience to stress as well as supporting recovery.

The Berlin Aging Study, involving several hundred people aged between 61 and 82, suggests that living in proximity to forest areas is linked with stronger, healthier functioning of the amygdalae, and the ability to better cope with stress as a result. While this association does not prove causality, there is growing evidence that spending time in nature, specifically wooded areas, is good for your health.

Stanford research, which involved scanning the brains of participants before and after a 90-minute walk, found that those who walked in nature as opposed to an urban street showed reduced levels of activity in an area of the brain linked to depressive rumination – the subgenual prefrontal cortex[37]. Based on their own subjective feedback, the nature walkers also became less self-critical. As you quieten your inner critic, that inner negative voice which replays all sorts of negative scenarios in your mind, you become nicer to yourself.

In Korea, FMRI scans were used by researchers to analyse brain activity in people who were looking at computer-generated images of either nature or urban areas. Those viewing the urban images had increased blood flow in the brain's amygdalae, implying higher levels of stress and anxiety[38]. On the other hand, those viewing nature scenes lit up those brain areas that support empathy and altruism – the anterior cingulate gyrus and insula.

Recent research from Denmark has found that exposure to nature can improve long-term mental health[39]. Irrespective of degree of affluence, social standing or family history, there was a 55 per cent variation in the prevalence of mental health conditions from the least green to most green areas.

Voluntary attention is the conscious use of attention to cope with the busyness of being out there in the world – for example, driving the car, dealing with traffic lights, etc. This leads to the rapid onset of mental fatigue and impaired focus, as the brain gets tired after prolonged usage and particularly with distraction. Through a process known as Attention Restoration Theory, it has been discovered that even a short exposure to nature can help the brain recover and restore its inherent ability to direct attention. This builds attentive focus and enhances your ability to persist with challenging problems for longer. Involuntary attention, on the other hand, also called soft fascination, requires no mental effort at all, and just happens naturally. This is what you use as you experience the sights, sounds and sensations of nature, gently restoring your mental clarity and ability to think more clearly, boosting reflection as well as allowing your mind to wander.

The 'forgotten antibiotics' of fresh air and natural light were espoused as far back as 1859 by Florence Nightingale's *Notes on Nursing*: 'Little as we know about the way in which we are affected by form, by colour and light, we do know this, that they have an actual physical effect.'

Being outdoors in nature boosts positive emotions such as contentment, gratitude and appreciation, among others. At a neurochemical level, time in nature can enhance levels of positivity hormones, including serotonin, oxytocin and dopamine – all elements of the 'Magnificent Seven' that I mentioned previously – leading to feelings of calm positivity. These positive emotions in turn 'broaden and build'. In other words, they widen (broaden) your attention span and enhance (build) the amount of material that you can stay focused on at any one time. This can be hugely beneficial for creative problem solving and maintaining a wide perspective on challenging complex ideas and problems. As positive emotions also help build social relationships, this can further support collaboration and crossover of support and ideas. The net effect of this is that by gifting yourself more time in nature, you can feel more creative, confident and connected to the world around you.

THE BENEFITS OF NATURE

Psychologists have found an interesting correlation between nature, openness and **creativity**[40]. Being in nature boosts your openness to experience, which in turn builds creativity and can support your happiness. It's not just green spaces either – the yin and yang of interconnection means that decluttering your own outer environments helps you to declutter and destress on the inside. Cultivating, creating and caring for the physical space of your garden can help clear the inner space of your mind. Nature's creativity feeds your own creativity, just as nature's essence fuels your essence. Planting seeds leads to fresh growth, not just of plants, but of new ideas, hope and possibility. Time in nature can bring on a state of flow, enabling you to think, feel and simply be closer to your creative best.

Sometimes known as the 'sixth sense', **awe** is a fascinating emotion with tremendous benefits on overall wellbeing and vitality. Awe allows you to step outside of yourself. Spending time in nature can boost feelings of awe, wonder and transcendence, feeling part of something bigger than yourself. Furthermore (and possibly unique among positive emotions), feelings of awe can lower levels of an inflammatory marker called interleukin 6 (IL-6)[41].

Nature can **inspire** and connect you with your higher power. It can take your breath away, sharpening your focus, brain functioning and critical thinking abilities. It can significantly change your self-perception, known as the 'small self' effect, as you feel smaller and less significant in relation to the world around you. Awe can act as a significant buffer against financial and other everyday stressors. It supports mindful presence, which may expand perceptions of time and counteract feelings of time pressure. As feelings of stress are alleviated, you boost your mood, wellbeing and overall sense of life satisfaction.

Being in nature exposes you to **natural light** which is a tremendous way to reset your circadian rhythm (your own natural body clock). So much time is spent indoors on screens now that for many people their body clock is out of sync. Lux is simply a measurement of light intensity. Spending time indoors in the typical office or home exposes you typically to less than five hundred lux. A sunny day outdoors can provide exposure up to 100,000 lux (perhaps up to 25,000 lux in the shade). Even an overcast day can provide at least 1,000 lux, and exposure of at least 30 minutes a day supports emotional vitality. Morning light with its blue tinge and shorter wavelength appears to be best. Even in wintertime, getting outdoors for a walk during lunch has significant health benefits as the outdoor light is always stronger, brighter and so much better for you than indoor artificial light.

IN MY PRACTICE

Melissa had been going through a particularly difficult time in her life when she attended me in my medical practice. Multiple life stressors, including dependent elderly parents, extra pressure at work and a recent health scare, were taking their toll. She felt irritable and short-fused, under constant time pressure and with a general sense of life 'speeding up'. Melissa's self-care strategies had understandably fallen by the wayside, as often happens with those suffering from negative aspects of stress.

Melissa understood that, while she couldn't change the situational stressors in her life, she could change how she saw things. At my suggestion, she went for some talk therapy (counselling), which helped her to see things differently.

She also recognised the importance of making some positive lifestyle changes. We spoke about exercise and movement, and while Melissa was never an avid exerciser, she had seen me on a TV programme talking about forest therapy and had later read an article about the benefits of spending time in nature. This was something that interested Melissa as a good friend of hers had 'green fingers' and would walk with her.

I prescribed regular time in nature, at least 120 minutes over the course of a week with no upper limit. And not just time, but a focused immersion among the wonderful plants at the world-class Mount Congreve gardens.

Time in nature allowed Melissa to disconnect from the noise of everyday life and to reconnect with a sense of stillness, the essence of who she was. I suggested that she write down her worries in a notebook before going out, and then to really let go of them during the nature walk. While in nature, Melissa was encouraged to absorb her experiences. The sounds (birdsong, wind rustling, leaves shifting underfoot) that she could hear; the sights (speckled sunlight, distant horizons, the fractal patterns or finer details in a leaf) that she could see; the smell of the fresh forest fragrance and the feel of the breeze against her cheeks or the sun at her back. Afterwards,

Melissa would write a few lines detailing how she felt, along with a simple expression of gratitude for the experience.

I met Melissa again about eight weeks later. She felt much better. Her mood had lifted, and her stress symptoms had largely abated. The improvements are perhaps best summed up in her own words: 'I started the nature time with an open mind, but I had no idea how much it would benefit me. It has made me feel a lot less irritable and stressed, and far more connected to the world around me. The forest therapy exercises give me such a sense of peace and stillness. I feel calmer, much more grounded and, dare I say, content. Time has slowed down in that I'm more present, and there seems to be more time available to me now. I'm really looking forward to things again now and feel genuinely hopeful and positive for the future.'

THE NATURE PRESCRIPTION

I've always found something special about trees, from producing oxygen and purifying air to providing shelter and a safe space to recharge and reconnect. Not to mention their towering strength and sense of stillness as the wind rustles through the leaves. Now, there is a wealth of scientific data from around the world supporting nature's health and healing benefits. What started out as plain common sense has evolved to become a new paradigm for health, vigour and vitality. A medical doctor, Qing Li, was interested in treating the Japanese problem of *karoshi* or 'death from overwork', well recognised as affecting Japanese workers in their prime. He had been impressed by the personal benefits he had experienced by spending time in nature and began to conduct experiments on his patients to see if science could objectively back up his subjective opinions. Research began in Akasawa, one of the most fragrant forests in Japan with four clearly defined seasons.

His initial research found that time in nature (as little as two hours once a month) could significantly lower stress hormone levels while increasing feelings of vigour and vitality. By comparing urban walks with walks in forests at a leisurely pace, he found that forest walks subjectively improved mood and lowered anxiety, while enhancing sleep and energy. Within minutes of spending time in nature, heart rate and blood pressure can lower, followed by a reduction in cortisol levels after 20 to 30 minutes. Objective data showed lowering of cortisol levels (12 per cent), blood pressure (1.4 per cent), heart rate (6 per cent) and overall stress activity in the body[42].

Qing Li's next research question was: 'If nature reduces toxic stress, can nature increase natural killer cells?' Natural killer (NK) cells are white blood cells that form a key component of your immune system and help to protect you from unwanted invaders, including virally infected and tumour cells. Dr Li's research in Japan found that middle-aged Japanese businessmen who spent two hours hiking in the forest each day for three days significantly increased their levels of natural NK cell levels (by 40 per cent). This persisted for up to 30 days, at which time he found the levels to be still 15 per cent higher than at the start of his research. Furthermore, he found that people living in areas with more trees have significantly lower levels of stress and lower mortality rates.

This led to the adoption of the term 'forest bathing', or *shinrin-yoku* from the Japanese words *shinrin* meaning forest and *yoku* meaning bath. It's interesting to note that while walking and movement in general reduces feelings of anxiety and depression, only shinrin-yoku impacted positively on vigour and vitality.

In essence, shinrin-yoku is the practice of immersion in nature using your five senses of seeing, smelling, listening, touching and tasting. This enables you to connect in a more immersive manner with the natural world. By bathing in the essence of the forest and plugging into the natural rhythm of nature, you can recharge and relax in a way that supports harmony and healing. Let's explore how some aspects of shinrin-yoku can boost your health and vitality.

Sight: As a highly visual creature, you will perceive most of your world through your sense of sight. Blues and greens found in nature are the most calming and restorative colours. Photoreceptor pigment genes in your eyes are hardwired to recognise the wavelengths of light reflected from green plants. At a very basic level, the colour green implies the presence of water (therefore food is nearby!) so you can turn down the stress response and relax a little. University of Rochester research has found that simply looking at the colour green before a creative task is enough to boost actual creativity[43]. By contrast, the grey landscape of an urban scene has been found to increase aggression and unhappiness.

Komorebi is a Japanese term which translates roughly as 'the sunlight filtering through the leaves in the trees'. Dappled sunlight would be a close English equivalent. Komorebi is especially beautiful with a low sun or early morning fog, with patchy light delighting the senses. And have you ever noticed how pleasing patterns in nature can be? This is largely because of the health-boosting benefits of looking at fractals. First described by Polish-born mathematician Mandelbrot as the 'roughness' of the world, fractals are the complex and irregular geometric patterns that repeat at different scales (called self-similarity). While fractals are absent from the modern man-made environment, just open your eyes in nature and you can experience engaging fractal patterns all around you. Look at the unfurling petals of a flower, the leaves of a plant and the division of a tree into its ever-smaller branches. Notice how the pattern of the branches remains the same no matter what scale you observe it from. Consider clouds, cauliflowers, coastlines – they all follow a fractal pattern. Furthermore, the retina in the eye appears to have a search pattern to rapidly recognise and resonate with fractal patterns, enabling the brain to make rapid decisions from an array of sensory data and stimulation. The brain appears to be hardwired to seek out and be visually fluent in these fractal patterns of nature, finding them inherently pleasing, naturally destressing and powerfully restorative. This is one of the key reasons why scenes of nature provide such a sense of restorative recharge, relaxing you while boosting wellbeing, feelings of awe and inspiration.

Roger Ulrich, an American professor of healthcare design and environmental psychologist, has found that merely looking at a scene from nature can significantly lower the stress response (physiologically and psychologically) and promote healing. As a young man, he suffered from kidney problems which required him to spend long periods of time bedbound at home. He had a view of a beautiful tree from his bedroom window which he felt raised his spirits. Years later, he wondered whether the same benefits might apply to patients in hospital. To further this question, he studied two groups of patients recovering from gallbladder surgery. One group looked out from their room at a brick wall, while the other group looked at trees. He found that those patients whose room looked out at trees recovered more quickly after the procedure, spent on average a day less in hospital, needed less pain medication and were less depressed with lower levels of stress, with far fewer negative comments being recorded in the nurses' notes. This research became the basis of his now-famous paper published in 1984: 'View through a window may influence recovery from surgery'. Replicated many times since, this research shows that people who benefit from a 'green view' have shorter hospital stays and require less medication than those who don't. Follow-up research in the University of Kansas suggests that it is the view of nature in particular, as opposed to other forms of distraction such as a television screen, that provides the healing benefits. Furthermore, the presence of plants and flowers in a healthcare setting provides evidence of a well-cared-for place, which in and of itself has a benefit, leading to the release of endogenous endorphins which are natural pain killers as well as providing positivity and calm optimism.

Sound: When was the last time you heard nothing? The Olympic National Park in Washington state has a small red stone that marks 'one square inch of silence' to represent the idea of creating a place completely free from man-made noise. Traffic, technology and the turmoil of modern life can all create a lot of noise, which can be stressful, impacting sleep and raising blood pressure. The stillness of the forest can boost what's termed cognitive quiet, which bathes your brain in silence for sensual vitality. John Ruskin wrote: 'No air is sweet that is silent; it is only sweet when full of low currents of under sound-triplets of birds, and murmur and chirps of insects.' Natural soundscapes from nature can be so tranquil, reducing the stress response and plugging you into restorative recharge. Birdsong has been shown to boost mood and mental alertness as well as build connection and a sense of serenity. Listen to the sounds of nature – water, wind and particularly birdsong – and notice how you feel.

Smell: Petrichor is the name given to the wonderful forest aroma experienced after it has rained. The word means the essence of rock or the smell of life and comes from the Greek *petros*, 'stone', and *ichor*, 'the vital essence that flows in the veins of the gods'. As the most primal sense, with a direct effect on body and mind, smell can powerfully affect mood and evoke visceral memories. Geosmin is the (usually pleasing) aroma of wet soil due to the effect of soil bacteria which also gives root vegetables and carrots their earthy taste. Humans are extremely sensitive to geosmin, which may be detected at levels of as little as five parts per trillion. In ancestral times, this sensitivity was thought to support the search for and detection of food, especially after a period of drought. Mycobacterium vaccae, a family of bacteria that lives naturally in soil (especially when the soil is enriched with manure or compost), boosts serotonin levels when inhaled or ingested while digging and weeding the garden. Breathing this in can boost subjective feelings of happiness and wellbeing, while dissipating worry and negative thoughts.

Trees connect, communicate and collaborate to collectively support each other and defend themselves against infestation with viruses, bacteria and fungi. They do this – through a network sometimes known as the wood wide web – by releasing substances known as phytoncides. The word 'phytoncide' comes from the Greek words *phyton* and *cide* (meaning 'plant' and 'to kill'). Trees such as pines, cypress, conifers and other evergreens are the largest producers of phytoncides. In addition, the environment around trees is also oxygen-laden, in addition to being rich in these health-enhancing healing properties of plants.

Taste: Open your mouth to taste the fresh woodland air or falling raindrops. Bringing some fresh strawberries along with you can provide for a wonderful sensual treat. Alternatively, bring a raisin or two with you to experience a simple mindfulness technique based on the simplicity of a raisin. Developed by Jon Kabat-Zinn, it not only supports mindfulness in general but more mindful eating. It enables you to savour and more fully experience the present moment, to be less distracted by the dizziness of everyday life and the 'merry-go-mind' of anxious negative thoughts.

○ Take a raisin and **hold** it either between your thumb and index finger or in the palm of your hand.

○ Pretend you've never **seen** anything like this before. Pay attention to the raisin and look at it carefully. Examine the ridges, asymmetries, areas that are lighter or darker in colour. Observe any features that are unique to it.

○ Roll the raisin carefully between your fingers to **appreciate** the texture. Perhaps do this with your eyes closed to better hone in on your sense of touch.

○ Hold the raisin beneath your nose and inhale the aroma or **smell**. Have you experienced this smell before?

○ **Place** the raisin at your lips and then into your mouth. Become aware of the sensations of having it in your mouth, exploring the raisin with your tongue, without chewing or biting on it.

○ Chew the raisin slowly and deliberately as you experience the emerging **taste**. Focus your awareness on the changing nature of the raisin as you chew mindfully.

○ Become aware of the desire to **swallow** the raisin and stay present as you swallow it.

○ Turn your awareness to the swallowed raisin as it moves

towards your stomach before tuning into how you now **feel**.

○   One small raisin can represent your choice to be more present, gifting you freedom from toxic stress with more peace and positive emotion, deepening your sensual immersion in nature.

Touch: Ions are particles present in the air which may be positively or negatively charged. Negatively charged ions are thought to have restorative benefits, for energy, clarity and overall vitality. They are much more prevalent outdoors and particularly prominent in forests and near waterfalls, rivers and streams. For example, a waterfall may contain up to one hundred thousand negative ions per cubic centimetre compared with a few hundred in your office at work.

Consider the earth as being like an enormous battery that grounds or earths you. Removing your shoes and walking bare-footed can enable you to become grounded with the electrical energy of the earth. Experience it for yourself and see how good it can feel to energise yourself in this way. Shoes made from leather help to maintain a natural connection with the earth, whereas rubber-soled shoes insulate you from the earth's natural flow.

Simply pay attention to the nature that's already in your life, whether an indoor plant, scene from your window or a walk in the local park. Becoming aware of the many positive emotions triggered by nature can further enhance and strengthen them. Something I love to do is to take a photo of a beautiful nature scene that captures my attention. Later on, I write a few lines to capture why I took that particular photograph and the feelings the image evoked. Taking time to review these descriptive photos becomes an ongoing conversation with the vitality-boosting benefits of engagement with nature.

If you are lucky enough to work near any green space, no matter how small, try to spend some time there regularly, perhaps during your lunchtime break. Every day in my medical practice, staff and patients alike are able to either spend time in the healing garden or simply enjoy its revitalising benefits by seeing it through the consultation room or cloister windows. Linking back to Ulrich's findings, research has found that a view of nature through a window can reduce work stress significantly and strengthen workplace positivity. More recently, the University of Melbourne has found that a short, green micro-break of a view of nature through a window lasting as little as 40 seconds can boost attention and alertness. If you are not fortunate enough to have that option at work, then consider a beautiful scene from nature as a screensaver on your computer or phone. University of Michigan research has found that simply looking at pictures of nature for 10 minutes can boost cognitive functioning.

Forest therapy (or bathing) is about your willingness to fully engage and be mindfully present during an immersive experience with nature. Mindful presence means exactly that – being mindful about being present. In other words, being where you are when you're there, fully and completely. As a practice, while a couple of hours is optimal, even 45 minutes will be enough time to enhance your vitality. Forest therapy is an opportunity to disconnect your mind from the busyness and distraction of everyday life, to reconnect with nature and the essence of who you are. (This isn't possible if your phone is buzzing in your back pocket, so leave it at home, turn it off or place it on silent mode.) Disconnect and let go of concerns about the stresses and strains of life while you immerse yourself in nature. As an idea, you could 'park them' by writing them down in a notebook or journal before you start. If there is some issue you want to solve, set a simple intention as you begin your immersion in nature. Let it go and allow your subconscious mind to get to work. Perhaps later in the day you will gain fresh insights or new perspectives.

Reconnect with how you feel. Firstly, find a relaxing place. Slow down and let your senses guide your body as you immerse yourself in the experience of nature and the richness of the natural world. Walk slowly to keep your senses attuned to your environment. Become one with nature, using your five senses of smell, sound, sight, touch and taste. If you like, sit down for a while and read as you simply imbibe and soak up the sounds, sensations and scenery around you. Give your analytical mind a brain break as you tune into your feelings. Simply notice what you notice, over and over again. Become the noticer of what you notice, the observer of all your experiences.

What do you **notice**? What are your eyes drawn to? What do you see? Different shades of green and the speckled sunlight? Fractal patterns from leaves in the trees or clouds in the sky? Can you see the patterns in the flower petals or the veins in a leaf? As you become more attuned to the unfolding fractal patterns that surround you, can you experience a sense of awe of the natural world?

What **sounds** can you hear and where is the source? Birds singing? The wind rustling gently through the trees? Twigs crunching underfoot?

What do you **smell**? The soil, plant aromas, phytoncides – or just rich, clean air?

What can you **taste**? Bringing along some fresh berries to eat can provide a wonderful immersive experience. Alternatively, just opening your mouth to taste the forest air (or rain) can further deepen your connection with nature.

What can you **touch**? How does your body feel as it moves? Put your hands on a tree trunk and feel its rugged presence. Hug it if you wish. Lift up some leaves or small stones. If appropriate, remove your socks and shoes to connect with the ground beneath you. Imagine roots spreading downwards from your feet into the ground as you plug into relaxation and recharge from stress.

Before you leave the natural space, reflect on all you have experienced. Consider writing a few lines in a journal or notebook. What did you experience? How do you feel now from an emotional viewpoint, compared to beforehand? Do you feel more relaxed and revitalised? How can this experience inform your life going forward? Ending with a simple gratitude practice helps to further consolidate the shinrin-yoku experience and deepen your relationship with nature.

One of my favourite descriptions of forest therapy was written by Helen Keller, who was blind. Her friend, who had just returned from a long walk in the woods, described 'nothing in particular' when asked what she had seen. In response to this description, Helen wrote:

I wondered how it was possible to walk for an hour through the woods and see nothing of note. I who cannot see find hundreds of things: the delicate symmetry of a leaf, the smooth skin of a silver birch, the rough, shaggy bark of a pine. I who am blind can give one hint to those who can see: use your eyes as if tomorrow you will have been stricken blind. Hear the music of voices, the songs of a bird, the mighty strains of an orchestra as if you would be stricken deaf tomorrow. Touch each object as if tomorrow your tactile sense would fail. Smell the perfume of flowers, taste with relish each morsel, as if tomorrow you could never taste or smell again. Make the most of every sense. Glory in all the facets and beauty which the world reveals to you.

The Mind of Vitality

The mind of vitality is resilient, focused and less prone to distraction. By taking a strength-based approach to life, you will learn to reframe your past experiences for growth and new perspectives. In this section I hope to help you see stress not as a threat to be thwarted or a symbol of superior capacity, but as something to be embraced. Recognising the importance of regular, restorative recharge from stress, you will actively engage with mindful practices to embrace present-moment awareness. And the mind of vitality never stops learning and growing. Small positive changes, consistently applied over time, can lead to big results.

Mindful presence

'You have power over your mind,
Not outside events.
Realise this, and you will find strength.'

MARCUS AURELIUS

Mindfulness has its origins in Buddhism, where the term *sati* (meaning attention, awareness and being present without judgement) was considered a first step towards enlightenment. Once viewed with suspicion, as a proxy promise for peace and tranquillity delivered from the depths of Buddhist temples, the practice has gained widespread acceptance in the Western world, thanks in large part to Jon Kabat-Zinn's mindfulness-based stress-reduction programmes at Massachusetts Medical School. In parallel, the scientific community has seen exponential growth in research studies showing quantum benefits when it comes to mindfulness and health – mental and emotional as well as physical.

THE SCIENCE OF PRESENCE

The ability to sit still and be fully present has never been more challenging, given the fast-paced nature of the modern world, with so much choice, clickbait and constant opportunity for digital distraction.

Noise pollution, particularly from urban living, increases the risk of high blood pressure, heart disease and can damage your hearing. So many people are experiencing information overload – data smog – from a mind-boggling array of sensory inputs – from the endless 24/7 news cycle to ever-present digital devices. All of this 'noise' leads to more toxic stress, mental fatigue, distraction, diminished focus and willpower.

I call this the **SPAM mind** – Syndrome of the Partially Attentive Mind – the sense that something 'out there' or 'in here' is always more interesting than what is right in front of you. Symptoms of the SPAM mind include mindless eating, forgetting someone's name as soon as you hear it, losing your keys, phone or credit card. Being so distracted by something that you forget to do something important right now. You get up in the morning and questions flood your brain as you grapple with an array of emails and social media notifications. What will I wear? What fires do I need to put out first at work? What will I eat first? This **paradox of excess choice** was eloquently articulated by Confucius, who wrote that the man who chases many rabbits catches none. So many people are submerged in a world that is always on, distracted by the era of obsessive hyperconnectivity, which contributes to the epidemic of anxiety and heightens the intensity of the stress response.

The SPAM mind is heightened by distraction and overload from digital devices, with a potential detrimental impact on your mental health. I call them potential weapons of mass distraction, leading to a deficit in attention from a constant ping in your inbox. Distraction keeps you chained to the shallow surface of the mind. Research suggests that as the brain grows dependent on phone technology, the intellect can weaken. I recall a senior executive recently admitting to me a compulsion to check his Twitter notifications in the midst of team leadership meetings! He's clearly not alone, as recent Ofcom UK research found that people on average:

○ Check their smartphone every 12 minutes, more than 80 times a day

○ Check their smartphone within 5 minutes of waking up – 40% of people (65% for 18–34-year-olds)

○ Check their smartphone within 5 minutes of turning the light out – 40% of people (60% for < 35-year-olds)

○ Spend 2.5 hours a day on their smartphone (3.25 hours for 18–24-year-olds)

The smartphone is a really powerful psychoactive substance, providing variable rewards with neurobiological reinforcement via the activation of dopamine pathways in your prefrontal cortex. This dopamine release can trigger feelings of compulsion and addiction. Time distortion, disinhibition, ease of access and perceived anonymity all combine to provide a perfect tool for digital distraction.

With many competing demands for your attention and energy, there is an inevitable tendency to **multitask**. Stanford University research has found that multitasking is often counterproductive, in that trying to do many things at once often means doing next to nothing at all[44]. Multitasking is perhaps better termed 'switch tasking', as your brain switches attention rapidly from one task to the next. The brain's bandwidth of active cognitive capacity is limited to dealing with just a few chunks of data at any one time (seven chunks, in fact, plus or minus two). Rapid switching over and back, from one task to the next, burns valuable brain energy and may reduce brain efficiency by up to 40 per cent.

Research has found that you are likely to experience upwards of 6,000 (mostly negative) thoughts today, with many of these the same thoughts as those you had yesterday (and the day before)[45]. At any given moment, your brain can receive about 11 million pieces of information, while you are only consciously aware of about 50 of them. The electrochemical pathways in your brain deliver thoughts seconds ahead of you becoming consciously aware of them.

While you have many thoughts each day, you are not your thoughts. Thoughts come and go like leaves in the wind. Just as you can't control what leaves blow into your garden, you can't control your thoughts. But you can choose to rake and weed your garden, just as you can choose what thoughts to focus your attentive awareness on. The trouble with all these thoughts is you can believe they are true, leading to depressive ruminations, feelings of anxiety and toxic stress. Rather than the present, you tend to focus on the past (regret, setbacks, disappointments) and future (stress, worry and anxiety) in the endless movie that is your life.

Not being able to quieten these thoughts at night can lead to disrupted sleep, where you are tired but wired. Furthermore, you may end up spending most of your time literally living in your own head. This 'merry-go-mind' craves distraction. So, when smartphones arrived, digital dependency from the SPAM mind met the magnetic attraction of the digital device.

This was a lesson well learned by me in late 2013, when I was taking night-time refuge in my mobile phone. So much distraction, so many apps a mere fingertip away. Of course, the alarm clock function was just the perfect excuse to bring it to bed, where last-minute emails could be drafted or read. First thing in the morning, I was straight onto the news (almost invariably bad news) and emails, before I even got out of bed. As I began to apply the techniques of mindfulness in my own life, it was far easier to understand that phones late at night just didn't cut the mustard. Of course, learning more about the emerging science of sleep and the deleterious impact of blue wavelength light was a great help. No more late-night technology – I began to park the phone safely in its docking station in the kitchen at an appropriate wind-down time. The results: my sleep quality improved, I felt sharper, better able to focus my attention, less anxious and less stressed. This one simple positive habit change had a cascading overall benefit.

Research from Harvard Medical School on the area of neuroplasticity has found that an eight-week mindfulness programme can begin to 'rewire' your brain. Specifically, the brain volume and grey matter increase in the hippocampus (an area of the brain involved in learning, memory storage, spatial orientation and encoding emotional context from the amygdalae) and the temporoparietal junction (an area involved in empathy and compassion). Furthermore, the density of the amygdala decreases, reducing the tendency to react to toxic stress (less fight or flight).

THE BENEFITS OF PRESENCE

Mindful presence allows you to break the connection between past and future while opening up the potential of the present moment. Mindful presence enables you to see things as they really are, to tune in and appreciate your senses, to be fully present, here and now in this moment as you are reading this.

Imagine a jam jar filled with water. Take a large spoon of dirt, put it into the jar, put the lid back on and give the jar a good shake. The jar of water symbolises the mind, while the cloudiness and moving pieces of dirt represent your 'merry-go-mind' of noise, distraction and everyday challenging life events. Now, place the jar on a table and wait for the dirt to settle at the bottom. The settled jar represents mindful presence, as you rest in awareness with a newfound freedom to experience reality as it really is. You see the whole picture with more clarity: the clear water as well as the mud at the bottom.

Mindfulness is this awareness that arises from paying attention on purpose, in the present moment and non-judgementally. Imagine the curtains are closed in your bedroom, with a beautiful bright day beckoning outside. Mindfulness is opening the curtains to let the light in and reveal the beauty of the present moment. By lifting the veil on the past and the anxiety of the future, you are able to experience more clearly the reality of the present moment. The paying attention itself is more important than the specifics of what you are paying attention to.

Mindful presence is a way of being, an inner sense of balance that enables you to widen the bandwidth on the present moment. In so doing, you expand your capacity to learn and grow, express emotion and experience more fully the senses of touch, taste, smell, sight and sound.

Anxious negative thoughts (ANTs) and beliefs that are emotionally exhausting (BEEs) can become part and parcel of the merry-go-mind. They manifest in all sorts of ways – from all the recycled ruminations of should do, could do and must do, to the litany of excuses and expectations. Comparing yourself negatively to others, focusing on what you have not or who you are not (gratitude deficiency), catastrophising about the future or seeing yourself as a victim of your circumstances. Overall, they diminish your sense of self. Little wonder that so many people are overwhelmed by the merry-go-mind and weighed down by these ANTs and BEEs. They result in the reptilian part of your brain taking charge, hardwiring feelings of toxic stress, exhaustion and anxiety. You react impulsively instead of responding thoughtfully, acting in self-defeating, recycled patterns ruled by negative emotions like fear.

Unfortunately, old habits die hard, so these beliefs and conditioned responses can be hard to change. However, it is possible. You can choose to change this experienced reality by stepping back and building your self-awareness through mindful presence. Mindful presence expands present-moment awareness, filtering out more of the ANTs and BEEs. You observe these thoughts and emotions as they rise and fall, without judging them or becoming subsumed by them.

Mindful presence is a gift as a keystone habit and commitment to your own self-care. As Jon Kabat-Zinn writes, 'In Asian languages, the word for "mind" and the word for "heart" are the same. So, if you're not hearing mindfulness in some deep way as heartfulness, you're not really understanding it. Compassion and kindness towards oneself are intrinsically woven into it. You could think of mindfulness as wise and affectionate attention.'

Mindful presence brings you to a place of **being**, where you are more aligned with your true nature, and the emotional essence of who you are. By this, I mean moving from what you know or do or have, to who you are! As you rest in being, your sense of identity changes from 'I am what I do or have' to who you are, attuned to your sense of purpose and inner freedom. Just by being, you become more creative and open to new possibilities. You develop your inner capacity to not only listen but hear, to not only see but observe.

Valuing includes empathy and compassion. Empathy is feeling what others are feeling and experiencing, while compassion is a desire to help and alleviate suffering which grows from the chamber of the heart. The Sanskrit word for compassion is *karuna* which is derived from the root *kr*, which implies action. Service to others may be considered to be compassion in action. Doing is sometimes called **karma**, when you 'do' from this preparation in alignment with being and valuing.

In recent years, there is growing recognition of the potential benefits of mindfulness to help address anxiety, face fears and combat toxic stress, thoughts and negative emotions. While mindfulness is certainly no panacea for all of your problems and life challenges, there are significant potential benefits.

Long-term mindfulness meditation can **quieten** this tendency of the merry-go-mind to make you 'get lost' in your own head as you ruminate endlessly about negative thoughts and experiences. This, of course, can be quite exhausting and energy depleting. Mindfulness moves you from stressing about what *has* happened (past) and/or worrying about what *might* happen (future) to what actually *is* happening (the present moment). You become empowered to run your own mind, rather than the merry-go-mind running you ragged.

Mindfulness or mindful presence can become a key strategy to strengthen your **sense of self** from self-awareness, self-acceptance and self-compassion to self-confidence and self-worth. In so doing, you deepen your connection to yourself and to the world around you. You become more of a leader in your own wellbeing as you become finely attuned to what's going on, rather than being a victim of circumstance or the vagaries of your merry-go-mind. As you strengthen self-control, you boost decision-making and think with more clarity, focus and perspective. Small, repeated positive changes add up over time to make a real discernible difference to the quality of your daily lived experience. Mindful presence supports self-understanding in terms of how thoughts and emotions impact your life. You are better attuned to your inner voice. Mindful presence supports self-care, as through your everyday actions you tell yourself 'I'm worth taking time out for.'

Mindfulness can reduce the inbuilt tendency to many forms of psychological bias, enabling you to see things as they really are, rather than as you think they are. It may well reduce negativity bias and enable you to become more aware of your **blind spots**. Not just blind spots about weaknesses or a self-sabotaging inner critic, but blind spots about your strengths and positive traits. Mindfulness broadens your worldview, enabling you to see multiple perspectives. Something I've often seen, which is a particularly 'Irish' trait, is someone who finds it hard to recognise a compliment, or who downplays or discounts its meaning immediately. Becoming more mindful enables you to better experience the positive.

Mindfulness helps to build connections within the vast array of brain networks, which improves the quality of your **attention** and reduces distraction. Working memory and willpower strengthen, in addition to self-regulation and brain changes that support impulse control. Mindfulness meditation builds your attentive awareness, which can have long-lasting improvements in attention span for up to five years after mindfulness training[46]. It enhances your ability to solve problems, while reducing mind-wandering. It can help reduce the tendency to stop paying attention to new information in your environment, known as habituation.

As you build more mindful presence, you boost your **confidence** to deal with challenging events, now and in the future. This enables you to build resilience and recharge from stress, not just from moment to moment, but on a longer-term basis.

Mental health improves as you become better able to **detach** from your thoughts or feelings, understanding that you are separate from them. This results in what's called 'freeing of the mind' (meta cognitive awareness). As you move from knowing to being, from past or future to the present moment, you reduce negative thoughts and dissolve anxiety (fewer ANTs). A mindful practice can become a helpful support for several mental health conditions including depression, anxiety and addiction.

Mindful presence may be considered an **emotional detox** that cools the amygdalae. Research from neuroscience has highlighted that mindfulness practices dampen down activity in the amygdalae (the emotional alarm centre or 'red button') in the brain and increase its connections to the prefrontal cortex (the logical thinking part of the brain)[47]. As a result, you become better able to manage and express emotions, less susceptible to the impact of negative emotions in others, less impulsive or reactive and more patient, responsive and resilient. It can be an effective coping strategy to cope better with uncomfortable emotions, rejection and social isolation.

Mindful presence can make **relationships** healthier as you become a better listener, get along at work more harmoniously, and appreciate others more. As you listen more to your inner voice, connecting with self-awareness and atunement, you experience more balance and harmony – I call this 'soulful presence'.

Mindful presence also promotes a more positive outlook on life in general and can support you to break old habits and build new, health-boosting habits. Being more mindful of your daily habits supports and motivates you to maintain more health-enhancing behaviours, including following a proper diet, getting adequate sleep and keeping up a regular exercise programme. Being mindful can improve sleep quality and reduce your tendency to insomnia. It can support the immune system and boost the brain's ability to process information (hippocampus), improving memory and reducing age-related problems. It can help with the management of chronic pain and improve quality of life. Overall, mindful presence is empowering, deepening your sense of wellbeing while enabling you to live more fully as you embrace each moment, one at a time.

THE MINDFULNESS PRESCRIPTION

Learning to become more mindful is something you must discover for yourself. Despite being such a simple, powerful tool, it remains undiscovered to most people. To help you adopt a more mindful approach to everyday life, here are some questions to consider as a starting point:

O   Are you stuck in your thoughts, reliving or recycling the past?

○ Are you living like a volunteer victim, criticising, complaining or negatively comparing?

○ Do you see your future in an open, positive and creative way?

○ Can you pay attention to what's going on at the present moment or are you distracted?

○ Do you suffer from entitlement or expectancy syndrome?

○ Do you crave approval from others or fear their criticism?

○ Can you listen well enough to hear what other people try to tell you?

Practise paying attention deliberately, for example, to the breath, to how your body feels – for example, your hands, your feet, your face – as you move your attention to one specific area at a time. Tune in to how you are feeling, paying attention to your feet on the ground, the chair you are sitting in, the sounds you are hearing – these are all ways to become more mindful.

Mindful silence: Try bathing your brain in silence for sensual vitality. Just think for a second: how many moments each day – if any – do you spend in total silence? Probably very few. If you're like most people, you spend your time in a world full of noise and rarely experience silence. As an experiment, stop what you're doing right now and listen. Listen hard. What do you hear? Try to identify every sound: traffic, computers whirring, music, people talking, your body, your breath.

Simply paying attention to the quality and quantity of sounds you hear can reduce noise-related stress and provide a wealth of benefits. What's more, with a dimension and quality all of its own, a daily dose of silence can help reset your inner thermostat to a state of more balance and harmony. For a final word on silence, here's the wisdom of monk Thich Nhat Hanh: 'Silence is essential. We need silence just as much as we need air. Just as much as plants need light. If our minds are crowded with words and thoughts, there is no space for us.' A daily dose of silence is a golden opportunity to disconnect from the technology and turmoil of the modern world and reconnect with the essence of who you are.

Of course, silence can be harmful if associated with loneliness, enforced disconnection from humanity (such as solitary confinement) or failing to speak out if struggling to cope or anxious. But what I'm talking about here is bringing mindful periods of silence into your everyday life. Even a few minutes in silence each day can be a real gift in allowing you to be more fully present. You can develop awareness of your thoughts as being mental processes that are not necessarily true and appreciate that they don't require you to take action or respond.

The restorative benefits of silence may be the complete opposite to the stressful effects of a noisy environment. Two minutes in silence may be even more relaxing for the brain than listening to 'relaxing' music, as measured by lowered blood pressure and increased blood flow to the brain. Time working in silence has been found to lessen cognitive load, reduce stress and support the alignment of your focus, attention and energy.

Periods of silence may even boost memory, with research on mice finding that spending two hours in silence each day led to the growth of new brain cells in areas of the brain linked to learning, memory and recall[48]. When I think of the benefits of silence, I'm reminded of Einstein's words: 'I think ninety-nine times and find nothing. I stop thinking, swim in silence and the truth comes to me.' Consider building some periods of silence into your day. Silence can be golden as a means to live with more vitality.

Mindful simplicity: Simplicity is a natural state of being. Mindful simplicity is your commitment to become aware of those things in your life that weigh you down with complexity, while taking active steps towards lightening the load and embracing inner freedom. Complexity can lead to emotional exhaustion, energy depletion and significant unhappiness. Examples of complexity include addiction, toxic relationships, unhealthy lifestyle habits and behaviour patterns. In a world of distraction, deadlines and so much stress, the problem with simplicity is that it can be so difficult to attain for so many.

Clutter and excess choice can compromise your ability to process information, stay productive and focus. Research from Princeton University has found that physical clutter competes for your attention (just like multitasking), reducing performance, productivity and ability to process information[49]. It acts like a restrictive straitjacket, sticking to the past, increasing stress and frustration with negative impacts on mood, while preventing you from experiencing creative insights or breakthroughs.

One of the great paradoxes of simplicity is that the mind craves both more *and* less. The ego craves newer, bigger, better in the belief that having more will relieve uncertainty and bring happiness. Any happiness gained, however, tends to be short-lived due to the psychological principle of adaptation. Newness and novelty can wear off pretty quickly as you adapt to your changed circumstances which become the new norm. On the other hand, particularly when you are under stress and feel overwhelmed, you often crave less to relieve stress, which in essence is a desire for peace. The essence of mindful simplicity for me means you don't need to have more, be smarter or better than anyone else. You just need to be yourself, tap into your true nature and open up to real presence, compassion and humility.

Here are some questions to consider:

○   What can you subtract from your life to enhance your wellbeing?

○   What can you stop doing?

○   What can you say no to?

○   Can you declutter – your spaces, your life?

○   Are you allowing others to clutter the spaces you share?

○   How complicated is your life right now?

○   Are you aware of just how much stuff you have accumulated?

○   How can you better use your time, spaces, thinking?

○   What can you release in terms of your beliefs or behaviours?

○   Have you fear of missing out (FOMO)?

○ Can you start to simplify?

○ Can you afford not to simplify?

Mindful simplicity lets go of attachment to possessions and moves towards simply being. Free from both materialism and fear of scarcity, you become kinder and more generous. Embrace mindful simplicity and begin to let go of some of the complexities and complications of life. Simplicity is an ongoing process that leads you to an inner place of security, serenity and stillness, a place where you feel content, grounded and at peace. In many ways, simplicity can be seen as a spiritual practice – connecting with the essence of your purpose and values – a habit of daily practice from the inside out.

Commit to starting. Give yourself a few minutes each day with the intention of clearing away complications. Simplicity is setting yourself free from the untamed ego, with its sense of expectancy and entitlement. Start with the smallest possible action you could take, then the next, and the next and so on. Simplicity is imperfect; it's all about progress. Over time, your consistency will build momentum and lead to big results. Enjoy the benefits of this 'ultimate sophistication'.

Mindful walking: Mindful walking has been espoused by many philosophers and deep thinkers through the ages from Wordsworth to Einstein. It sounds paradoxical; the idea of movement bringing you closer to peaceful presence and stillness. But the philosophy of mindful walking is simply to walk with full presence of body *and* mind, to be open and fully present to the experience. There is no point in walking through the woods while having a business call on your iPhone or while your mind is elsewhere. Put your phone away. Allow the pressing problems of your life to dissolve as you embrace the rich experience of nature. To experience the true benefits of mindful walking, walk effortlessly and immerse yourself fully in your environment. Listen to the sound of the wind rustling gently through the leaves. Hear the song that the birds sing. Inhale in the aromas of nature. See the real beauty around you. Look down at your feet. Experience the connection of touching the earth with your feet as you walk, free from worry, anxiety or distraction. Breathe in and breathe out. This is called Buddha-nature – full awareness of your surroundings. Reflect on who has taken this path before you, not yesterday or last week, but hundreds of years ago. As you engage fully with your surroundings, your mind is not empty or devoid of activity. Rather, the prefrontal cortex in your brain, the seat of thoughtful analysis, gets a well-deserved brain break, allowing you to move to a state of being.

Mindful eating: Be present when you eat. Give your full attention to what you are eating. Don't be distracted by your phone or thoughts of the day ahead. Stay present. When you eat, eat. Bring your full attention to this practice of eating. As your meal is there for you, so you have to be there for your meal. Eat with mindful presence. Enjoy each bite of food mindfully. Eat with gratitude. There is so much to be grateful for. The food itself. Those people that prepared the meal. The seeds that were planted and the crops that were grown. The earth that provided the crops. The sun and rain that helped the process. The Japanese tea ritual is an example of everyday mindfulness. Known as *Sado* or 'the way of tea' it is based on the timeless principle of *ichi-go ichi-e,* meaning one time, one meeting; for this time only, or to live each moment to the full as this may be the only day we have. It is a spiritual practice intended to bring peaceful equanimity through harmony with nature by preparing tea from the heart. It is based on the four principles of purity, tranquillity, harmony and respect. The symbolism of this tea ceremony is a great metaphor for the timeless principles of living fully and mindfully with simplicity, kindness and thoughtfulness.

Mindful moments: Mindful moments are mini meditative actions that last only for the duration of three breaths. Examples include wiggling your toes attentively, breathing slowly, feeling your fingertips or really seeing the person in front of you. These mindful moments build peaceful equanimity, self-awareness, curiosity, calm contentment and creativity. Stay present in other times too, such as when brushing your teeth. Enjoy the practice for the minute or two you have. Brush your teeth mindfully; don't be distracted by what's happening next. Be grateful for the practice, for having teeth to brush, for being able to take care of your teeth in this way. Here's a challenge for you. Do a hundred of these mindful moments each day for a week. My bet is that someone in your life who knows you well but isn't aware of your commitment will notice and comment on the change they have noticed in you.

Here's a simple exercise to help you become more mindful in everyday life.

o   List five things you can see.

o   List four things you can hear.

o   List three things you can feel.

o   List two things you can smell.

o   List one thing you can taste.

Mindful observing: Pick out something in your environment. It might be an object in your kitchen, a flower in your garden outdoors, or even the palm of your hand. Pay attention to this object. Look at it with curiosity, as if you are seeing it for the very first time. Notice the texture, the shape, the shadows, the undulations and contours.

Mindful gatha: A *gatha* – coming from the Sanskrit term for 'song' or 'poetic verse' – is a short expression of poetry or prose which is recited mentally (as opposed to out loud) in rhythm with the breath. It brings your attentive awareness more fully into the present moment as well as into the immediate future moment. The idea is to match alternate lines of the gatha with your inward and outward breath. Try this one:

Breathing in: I own my breath

Breathing out: I smile

Breathing in: I calm my body

Breathing out: I smile

Memorise four lines of a gatha that resonate with you.

Say them to yourself when you are engaged in a meaningful experience, for example, a walk in nature, hearing the birds sing or savouring your cup of coffee. As you repeat this practice, notice how you further deepen your sense of mindful presence and appreciation of the moment, in the moment.

Mindful breathing: When you were born into this world as a beautiful little baby, the first thing you did was to take a breath. And the last thing you will do in the world is draw your final breath. Breathing is essential to life itself, one of the most natural things to do as a human being. Breathing in brings oxygen, life and vitality to every cell in your body while breathing out expunges the body of waste material in the form of carbon dioxide. Normally, you breathe about 12 to 16 times a minute, without any effort or conscious awareness on your part. It's just something you do. While this process is under the automatic control of your autonomic brain, you can influence how quickly, deeply and deliberately you breathe. The easiest way to build more mindful presence is to notice when you aren't. When you feel stressed, anxious or distracted, simply embrace mindful presence, as you feel calm without effort or stress.

Allow yourself to take a **PAUSE**:

Pause: Take a pause from what you're doing for a moment.

Awareness: Become aware of how you're feeling right now in your body and mind. You may feel stressed or anxious. You may have tension in your shoulders.

Understand: Understand and appreciate that you are separate from the feelings you are experiencing. Imagine the river of life flowing in front of you. You are observing your feelings of tension and anxiety, understanding that you are separate from them.

Simply breathe: Take a big breath in from the top of your nose to the bottom of your lungs. Take a slight pause.

Exhale: Exhale through your nostrils all the way, slowly and steadily, until you empty your lungs. As you exhale, breathe out all your tension, toxic stress and feelings of anxiety. Let it all go, then take a slight pause at the end of your exhalation. Now repeat.

Take four to five of these breaths per minute for up to 10 minutes in total over the course of your entire day. Perhaps a couple of minutes on way to work, a minute or two before or after that important meeting or conference call, on the way home and a few minutes at night. In fact, slowing your breathing in bed can also help you relax your brain for a more restorative night's sleep. And it's such an easy thing to do – anywhere, anytime, with no special equipment or trip to the gym required! Taking a PAUSE quietens the stress response from the amygdalae (the emotional alarm centre), located close to the breathing centre in the brain. This dampens down and decreases feelings of anxiety or toxic stress, enabling you to feel emotionally more calm, cool and collected. It reduces feelings of being overwhelmed or emotional exhaustion.

Psychologically, intentionally slowing your breathing is a great reminder that you are in control, as you own and control your own breath. You gain clarity that you can focus your attentive awareness on the present moment, that instead of reacting, you can choose how to respond in any given moment. Mindful breathing can enable you to do just that, to live each moment with full attentive presence. As you focus your attentive awareness on the present moment, your mind becomes clearer and more engaged. By breaking the hold your hardwired emotional brain has on your mind, you can think more clearly and logically, you are less prone to distraction and make better decisions. Mindful breathing generates feelings of calm contentment which permeate the cells of your body and build a sense of inner peace.

Physiologically, the habit of regularly slowly your breathing increases heart rate variability (HRV). A higher HRV reflects more resilience to stress whereas research shows a connection between low HRV and worsening depression or anxiety[50]. Slowing your breathing builds inner connection, as breathing mindfully brings body and mind together as one. In many ways, the breath acts like a bridge between mind and body, finely tuning and closely integrating both. Mindful breathing builds overall connectivity, strengthening the mind–body, gut–brain and heart–brain connections.

Simply moving back to your breath also allows you to experience a deeper, richer connection with the world around you. To see different things and experience things differently. Mindful breathing can deepen and enhance your experience of your natural environment. As you spend time in nature with mindful breathing, you become more attuned to its vibrant sensuality. As you become more attuned to your breath, and your surrounding environment, you will experience a deep sense of relaxation and peace. Try a mindful breathing PAUSE as the sun rises, as the dappled sunlight appears through the leaves of a tree during a forest walk, as the waters of a stream flow gently by.

Finally, the word 'inspiration' comes from the Latin *in-spira*, meaning 'in spirit'. As you inspire, you breathe in and connect with your spirit and purpose. Becoming consciously aware of your breath in this way can become a valuable reminder of who you are and why you matter in the world. Adding in a short saying or mantra during the out breath can provide additional benefits, perhaps just a single word, like 'peace', the name of a loved one or some word that resonates meaning for you.

Mindful breathing is a wonderful reminder that you are here, not just for yourself but for those people that matter. As such, it is a key element of the energy required for effective self-care. How can you love yourself if you are not here? How can you care for anyone else if you're not here?

Overall, the PAUSE method of intentionally slowing your breathing has numerous potential benefits. It has to be one of the simplest and most effective habits to enhance your mindful presence and overall vitality. As you breathe more mindfully, you bring more of yourself into life. As you gift life with more of your presence, life will respond in kind by being here for you. This is the yin-yang of reciprocity. Try it out and see for yourself.

Mindful mundanity: Washing dishes is considered a pretty mundane task. As an experiment, people were split into two groups before washing dishes – one group read about mindful dishwashing while the other group read general information about cleaning dishes[51]. After the task, those who had been taught about mindful dishwashing experienced more mindful presence, more focused awareness of the task at hand, and felt more engaged, inspired and curious about the task itself.

Just think of the many daily activities that you currently do – most of them fairly mindlessly, like everyone else, I'm sure. Can you choose to carry out some of these tasks more mindfully with benefits for your wellbeing? Consider some of the activities we've touched on already – driving, brushing your teeth, walking, eating – and then reflect on how you might choose to carry these out through a more mindful approach. Are you mindful or is your mind full of ANTs or BEEs? Do you focus more on what you can or can't control?

Can you live more like a **lotus flower**? The lotus flower features prominently in many Eastern religions from Buddhism to Hinduism. It is a symbol of perfect balance, poise and peaceful equanimity. It doesn't need perfect conditions to start. Far from it: the lotus arises from the mud (dark, tough times) representing resilience. It floats gently on the water, symbolising simplicity, stillness and serenity. Rather than reaching high into the sky with an untamed ego that says 'look at me', it stays low and humble. It is content to let go of expectations. The lotus flower is attached to its sense of purpose and yet detached from the outer world. It is a great analogy for life itself – to let go of expectancy and entitlement and the vagaries of the untamed ego and simply be yourself. 'How can you be so beautiful and yet so humble? How can you be so powerful and yet so still? How can you be so inspiring to others and yet remain content to be yourself?' The lotus flower answers these questions. It simply is. It exists. It does its thing, mindfully. It espouses mindful presence. No fuss. No fanfare. Just a beautiful flower that needs nothing to remind it of how unique and beautiful it really is.

Just like you.

Mindful choice

'*Sickness is a hindrance to the body, but not to your ability to choose, unless that is your choice. Lameness is a hindrance to the leg, but not to your ability to choose. Say this to yourself with regard to everything that happens, then you will see such obstacles as hindrances to something else, but not to yourself.*'

EPICTETUS

Having started out in captivity as a Roman slave, Epictetus lived his life as a prolific exponent of Stoic resilience through his writings. Though he spent much of his life lame, lacking family or freedom, he fully accepted and made light of his situation. Through mindful choice, his mindset allowed him inner freedom, despite the slavery of his outer world. One of his key lessons is: 'Some things are up to us, and others are not.' Another is: 'It is the act of an ill-instructed man to blame others for his own bad condition.' The key idea is the appreciation of the crucial difference between those few things that are under your control and the many things that are not. For me, Epictetus's teachings provide a practical path to support you through the good and not-so-good times in life.

Which brings me to the idea of two circles: the circle of concern and the circle of control, each competing for your attention. Of course, where your attention goes, your energy flows.

The **circle of concern** represents the many things in life that you can't control or influence, yet which can captivate so much of your precious energy and attention. In the world of endless noise and digital distraction, it has never been easier to burn valuable attention, energy and time in this circle, resulting in even more ruminating worry and toxic stress. In the circle of concern, you may become a prisoner of the past – past regrets, failures and frustrations. A prisoner of your own thoughts and limiting beliefs, with the merry-go-mind of anxious negative thoughts. The circle of concern can drive negative thinking patterns, including perfectionism, expectancy, entitlement or endless excuses (which I term 'excuse-itis'). The circle of concern focuses on the flaws, failures and the 'what's wrong'. It can foster fear, aggravate anxiety and ramp up feelings of inadequacy, negative comparison and stress. Examples of the many, many things which may be in your circle of concern include the past, what other people think or say about you, other people's behaviour, the weather, the economy, the news, social media 'likes' and comments. Do you find yourself stuck in the past, on a treadmill or in a straitjacket of frustration? If so, are you spending too much time in your circle of concern?

Of course, there are important things in life that you should be concerned about. These include your health, your loved ones and important socio-political concerns of society. There are many things to be concerned about, and to pretend otherwise is delusional. Wellbeing is never about denying reality. However, it is important to not become disempowered by spending too much of your attentive awareness and valuable energy in this zone. Epictetus believed stress and unnecessary suffering arise whenever you try to exert absolute control over your circle of concern, which, of course, is impossible. Don't short-circuit your potential by being constrained here, expecting others or circumstances to change. Focus more on those things you can change and control, which brings me to the second circle.

In the **circle of control**, you choose to give more of your attentive awareness to those things you can control. Focusing on your circle of control enables you to make peace with your past, to let go and let be. To understand that everything you have learned up to now can be filed under 'research and development'. To live more in the present moment, embrace change and exert mindful choice over your actions and decisions. The circle of control helps you to gain courage and confidence from every experience; to appreciate that courage is not the absence of fear but the willingness to walk through your fears in pursuit of something that's important to you.

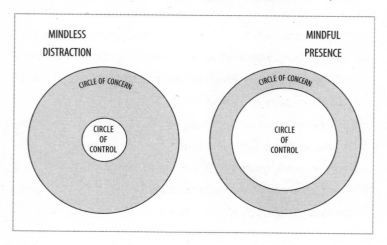

Are you more of a thermometer or a thermostat? A thermometer reacts to the temperature of its surrounding environment. It is the perfect metaphor for your circle of concern, always *reacting* to the temperature of events; to your inner world of thought and emotion, as well as to your outer world of experience. By contrast, the thermostat is pre-set to maintain a certain temperature, regardless of what's happening in the outside world. If you focus on your circle of control, your inner climate stays constant, no matter what your outer weather!

As a reminder, here are some things you actually **can** control:

O   Attitude and mindset
O   Strengths and values
O   Stress recovery and recharge
O   Thoughts you pay attention to
O   Self-talk
O   Letting go and forgiveness
O   Media exposure (mainstream and social)
O   Books you read
O   Commitment to self-development and learning
O   Self-care habits: exercise and movement, sleep quality and quantity, nutrition
O   Kindness and compassion
O   Gratitude and appreciation
O   People you reach out to and connect with
O   Mindful practices and meditation
O   Living with vitality

As you spend more time in the circle of control, you diminish your circle of concern as your circle of control gets bigger. In essence, you learn to choose how to respond and in so doing to exert more mindful choice. You accept some aspects of your circle of concern and appreciate the difference between these two circles. Epictetus's teachings provide a reminder not to become upset, frustrated or to waste energy on those things you cannot control. Instead, to let go and practise acceptance. To take responsibility for your circle of control – your thoughts and beliefs – as opposed to blaming others or abdicating responsibility. This is the idea of personal 'response-ability' – your ability to respond.

I mentioned Einstein's theory of the friendly versus hostile universe earlier – that if you believe you live in a friendly universe, you will act accordingly and actively seek evidence to support your worldview. However, if you believe you live in a hostile universe, more of this will show up in your circle of concern and in your life. By all means, do what you can to improve yourself and the world. At the same time, recognise the limitations of what you can and can't change. While you always have control and influence over your own actions and responses, you may have very little control over anything else.

As a doctor, I meet many people who struggle with the idea of 'letting go'. At times, this is perfectly understandable – letting go can be one of the most difficult things to do in life. At the same time, it can be incredibly energising and liberating. Counselling or **talk therapy**, particularly cognitive behavioural therapy with a suitably trained therapist, can support you to see things differently. As such, it can be invaluable if you are suffering from mood disorders, the merry-go-mind of anxious negative thoughts, or simply feel stuck in some aspect of your life. To let go and let be. To learn to let go of pain from the past or anxieties about the future. To let go of toxic stressors or negative noise in the world, of the need to micromanage others or control events. Instead, focusing on your mindful choice to be more present in the world; choosing to move from your circle of concern to your circle of control.

Analysis of wisdom books down through the ages, from the writings of Aristotle and Confucius to the Bible, Bhagavadgita and the Koran, suggests that there appear to be six core characteristics or virtues in common to every culture and religion, namely: courage, justice, humanity, temperance, transcendence and wisdom. These have been further subdivided into 24 character strengths, as shown in the list below.

o   **Courage:** bravery, perseverance, honesty, zest
o   **Justice:** leadership, fairness, accountability, equality
o   **Humanity:** love, kindness, social intelligence, community
o   **Temperance:** prudence, humility, self-regulation, forgiveness
o   **Transcendence:** spirituality, humour, gratitude, hope
o   **Wisdom:** curiosity, creativity, love of learning, perspective

These 24 strengths are uniquely arranged and configured in each person, resulting in your unique character profile and personal identity. While you have the potential to express all of these strengths, your unique mix helps to make you the person you are. Of course, your strengths can change over time and there are many ways to use them. As an analogy, you have lines in your fingers which are arranged uniquely as your unique fingerprint. Most people have several key strengths that they most easily identify with, that energise and excite them, that feel part of their real authentic selves. These are called **signature strengths**. But do you focus on your weaknesses as opposed to your strengths? On what's wrong as opposed to what's strong? If so, that's perfectly understandable, as your brain is hardwired to detect fear, anxiety and avoid discomfort in the primary goal of survival. Learning to focus on your strengths might feel counterintuitive as the reality is that most people tend to focus on their faults and flaws. Furthermore, taking your strengths and accomplishments for granted is common, as is the tendency to compare yourself less than favourably to other people who are stronger than you in a specific area.

Think of a beautiful swan, gracefully appearing to glide effortlessly on a lake. While others see the swan as a symbol of strength and serenity, the swan herself may be blind to this as she paddles her feet frantically beneath the surface to keep going, completely unaware of the strength others perceive. What's readily apparent to others may be a blind spot for you. If you're like many people, you may not even know what your strengths are. To reap the many benefits of choosing to live through a strengths-based mindset, firstly, you need to know what your strengths are and, secondly, learn to apply them in meaningful ways. Choosing what's strong over what's wrong has significant benefits for your overall vitality and ability to flourish. Look at the list of character strengths again. You can identify which are signature strengths for you if you answer 'yes' to the following questions. When you think of this specific strength, are you:

○   Energised and engaged using it?
○   Engaging with the essence of who you are, part of the 'real you' or authentic self?
○   Excited to use it, especially early on?
○   Enthused and experiencing positive emotion when using it?
○   Exploring ideas that revolve around it?
○   Experiencing a learning curve when you first practise it?
○   Encouraged by using it?

A strengths-based approach to life will make you mentally stronger, allowing you to do more and be more. It builds resilience, enabling you to cope more effectively with stress. Strengths support you to reframe challenging experiences through the lens of growth, a mindset change from hopeless to hopeful in the face of life's challenges, to mindfully choose what's strong as opposed to what's wrong. As you develop more awareness, clarity and insight into your innate strengths and abilities, you become better equipped to move forward with autonomy, self-acceptance and make real progress towards your goals.

Imagine a sailboat on the ocean which has a large sail and a leak: this leak, signifying key weaknesses, has to be plugged so the boat doesn't sink. However, if you just focus all your attention and energy on the leak, while you won't sink, you won't get anywhere fast. The big sail represents your strengths, which are essential to build resilience, overcome adversity and become a better version of you in the world. It is only by choosing your strengths that you will sail the ocean of possibility in your life.

Using your signature strengths regularly can significantly enhance your happiness and wellbeing, while lowering feelings of depression, with benefits lasting up to six months. Strengths can boost engagement, productivity and job satisfaction. Strengths shown to be particularly closely linked with your happiness and wellbeing include gratitude, hope (optimism), love, curiosity, enthusiasm, and, of course, strong interpersonal relationships.

For example, the strength of curiosity encourages you to explore what's novel about any situation, leading to new discoveries and personal growth. To build your strength of curiosity, you might decide to read an article or watch a documentary about something you know nothing about. You might talk to unusual people, expose yourself to new experiences and try new things. One of the best ways to build your curiosity is to study how young children interact with their environment, seeing the world through eyes of wonder, living more out of their imagination than their memory. Pablo

Picasso wrote that it took him four years to paint like Raphael but a lifetime to paint like a child; that every child is an artist, but the challenge is how to remain an artist and child-like when grown up!

Take a closer look at the strengths that you identified on page 266, and your own understanding of them, through the following questions:

O   Are you aware of your strengths?
O   Which aspects of everyday life enable you to use more of your strengths?
O   Which aspects drain you of your strengths?
O   Using which of your strengths enable you to become more fully alive?
O   Name a key strength in your life.
O   Who are the role models for the strengths you want to copy and emulate? Perhaps Martin Luther King Jr, for bravery and leadership, or Mother Teresa for love.

Now try looking at one particular strength that you identify with in terms of the past, present and future.

O   **Past**: Think of a time and situation in the past when you successfully used this strength.
O   **Present**: What does this strength look like right now in your actions, thoughts and conversations?
O   **Future**: How can you redesign your life so that you can better use this strength?
O   Why is it important to build this strength into your life?

O   What might the benefits be?

O   What's the one small step you can take today to start using this strength more in your life? If your strength is kindness, for example, can you commit to spend some time volunteering?

Choosing your responses

'I've learned that people will forget what you said, people will forget what you did, but people will never forget how you made them feel.'

MAYA ANGELOU

When it comes to your relationships, celebration trumps conflict. What I mean by this is that how you choose to celebrate and recognise the 'good news' that others share can make a big difference in terms of developing the quality of that relationship. This may include a hard-won promotion at work, a personal achievement or even a small incidental 'win' in the journey of life.

Research by Professor Shelly Gable has found that there are four ways of responding when someone shares a good news story or experience with you[52]. These four ways are described below.

Active and constructive

○ Verbal: High energy. Encouraging, enthusiastic, engaged, excited to learn more. Authentically and actively responds. Asks thoughtful questions that enable the person to share more details, to almost relive and re-experience the moment. Demonstrates empathy, understanding, value, connection, respect, interest, curiosity.

o   Non-verbal: Positive body language, eye contact, genuinely smiling, leaning into the conversation.

o   Example: 'That's terrific news, really great for you. Very well done. I'm so proud of you. I know this is important. Tell me how you felt when you first found out. What did you think? How are you going to celebrate?'

Passive and constructive

o   Verbal: Low energy, semi-interested but little enthusiasm expressed. Downplays the significance. Little emotional expression.

o   Non-verbal: Flat, not engaged or enthusiastic. Some support offered, perhaps a slight smile, but in a low-energy way, perhaps distracted by a phone, etc.

o   Example: 'That's nice. Good for you.'

Active and destructive

o   Verbal: Expresses negativity and actively highlights the downsides of this 'good' news. Downplays. Displays uncertainty and concern. Devalues and acts as a 'damp squib' on any excitement.

o   Non-verbal: Frowning and furrowed brow, glares, aggressive and assertive.

o   Example: 'Are you crazy? Do you not realise how stressful that's going to be? That sounds like such a bad idea to me, so risky!'

Passive and destructive

o   Verbal: Dismissive, disruptive and inattentive,

deliberately ignores the news shared or changes topic of conversation. No acknowledgement.

o   Non-verbal: No eye contact, turns away, may look at watch or even leave the room.

o   Example: 'What are we having for the dinner? What time is it? Let me tell you how great I am!'

Only the first way – active and constructive responding – supports the building of a relationship. In fact, how you share and discuss 'good news' events is more indicative of a robust relationship than how you fight.

Of course, at times we all need someone to confide in, someone to give us honest advice and feedback. This can be really important to keep us on track, perhaps with important decisions at stake. However, when someone chooses to share some good and exciting news with you, your initial response can have a major impact on the quality and longevity of that relationship, for better and for worse. Active and constructive responding validates and recognises the other person in terms of what they are sharing, in addition to your relationship with them.

Also known as **capitalisation**, it is thought to be effective through encouraging the retelling and resharing of positive events. In the yin and yang of dynamic relationships, active, engaged listening (verbally and non-verbally) facilitates more dynamic speaking and interaction. As such, positive emotions are re-experienced, which reinforces memory and supports meaning. It enables you to share in the joy of another person, which can provide the spark to ignite a stronger relationship. It builds trust, closeness, likeability and relationship satisfaction. Benefits include more positive emotion, increased subjective wellbeing, validation, perceived self-control and enhanced self-esteem with reduced loneliness and depressive symptoms. There is less relationship conflict and a stronger sense of connection, which work to enhance overall wellbeing. Active and constructive responding is the most empowering way to respond to another person, in a way that benefits the wellbeing of the recipient, the giver and the quality of the relationship overall.

Of course, developing this skill is a habit. With time and plenty of practice, it can be learned and developed. Many of your responses in existing relationships are conditioned by your previous experiences, and how distracted or stressed you are at the time. As a result, they may, at times, be less than mindfully considered. Think about some of your recent experiences with others. What 'good news' has been shared with you? How have you responded? What might a more active and constructive response have looked like? By focusing on specific elements of your praise and support, see how your communication and relationships can strengthen over time. Choose to be more mindful in your interactions and choose more active and constructive responding.

Research pioneered at Stanford University (and replicated more than a hundred times since) has found that writing about your values is one of the most powerful psychological exercises you can do to better embrace stress and build resilience[53]. The study involved college students, heading home for winter break, who were tasked to keep a daily journal while at home. One group was asked to write about the **personal values** that were most important to them and to describe how their daily life events connected with those values. A second group was simply asked to write about **positive events** that happened during their days. After winter break, when the students returned to Stanford, it was found that those students who had written about their personal values were happier, healthier, had experienced fewer illnesses and overall had a better attitude than those students who had simply written about positive life experiences.

So why did this have such a beneficial impact on mental health, positive health choices, resilience and ability to recharge from stress? Writing about your personal values in your journal transforms your view of stressful life events from something to be endured to something that enables you to grow and deepen your sense of meaning. In other words, it connects your everyday events to a larger 'why'. It supports a mindset change from pessimism to more mindful optimism. You tend to stop avoidant behaviours like denial or procrastination and become better able to face challenging situations head on. You recognise that setbacks, while inevitable, are not permanent or personal to you and that things can improve through the power of your efforts. It supports you to better see your job or current stressor through the lenses of: How can I serve and support others? How can I use more of my signature strengths? How can I make a difference? In this way, for example, a busy teacher who values leadership can see their role as inspiring the next generation of young people, rather than simply feeling stressed by the time pressure of the syllabus, etc. In short, you tell yourself a different kind of story: one that allows you to not just survive but thrive in the face of stress.

What's fascinating about this research is how simply writing about your values for 10 minutes **once** (not once a day or week, just the once!) can lead to significant gains for you in terms of your ability to build resilience and better manage stress. Writing a letter to your future self in terms of what you value, what's important to you and how you view your life can support your good habits and choices while preventing bad ones. This future version of you connects with and aligns more closely with your values, supporting 'continuity of self'.

THE PRESCRIPTION OF YOUR STORY

Lao Tzu wrote: 'At the centre of your being you have the answer; you know who you are and you know what you want.' The nature versus nurture debate focuses on whether you are a product mainly of your genes or your upbringing – your genetic code or your Eircode! However, there is a third element that is often forgotten: the narrative or **story you tell yourself**. What are the stories you are telling yourself about your life right now? Are they all true? Does your life story need updating? Can you tell new stories about yourself and your world?

Joseph Campbell wrote that you are a hero in the journey that is your life. While the path is often challenging, with many obstacles to overcome, and the destination rarely clear, in the end the hero's adventure is simply the adventure of being alive. This can be a valuable lesson to learn. While you can't change your genes or upbringing, you are the author of your own life story. When you recall or remember a past event, your brain reconstitutes the memory from the various parts of the brain it has been stored in. Rather than simply pressing the 'play button' to replay the memory, it is reconstructed. In doing this, your memory may be highly influenced by your emotions and beliefs at the time of remembering.

Mindful choice enables you to change the story you tell yourself. One technique for doing this is grateful reframing. Think about an unpleasant experience or hurt from your past. A tough time, setback or disappointment. Now, try to focus on the positive aspects of this challenging experience. In other words, remember that you survived! You got through the bad job. You got over that relationship. You made it through the tough times and you found a way back. This process of recalling how things were then (as opposed to how they are now) sets up a sharp contrast in your mind. The mind thinks in terms of **counterfactuals**. The greater the change from what you expected, the stronger and more intense the emotional reaction may be. This counterfactual tendency can also explain why you may experience such pain if you lose something you have taken for granted.

As a result of this life event:

○   What things have happened that you became grateful for even though you weren't at the time itself? How have you benefitted and become better as a human being?

○   How has it helped you to better appreciate the important
       people and things in your life? How has this event helped
       put your life into perspective?

○   Can you appreciate that things right now could be so
       much worse? By comparing how things were then versus
       now, do you feel grateful? How much better is your life
       now? How little have you really got to complain about
       right now?

As you reframe experiences through a more grateful lens,
you reduce their unpleasant emotional impact with grateful
coping leading to more positive consequences of negative
events. Reframing through the lens of gratitude is neither
denying reality nor a form of superficial happy positivity. It
does realise your mindful choice to reframe setbacks through
the lens of purpose and meaning, to recast negative experiences
as positive shoots for gratitude and growth. In short, to tell
yourself a different story.

In *Man's Search for Meaning*, Victor Frankl describes one
man's struggle for survival in the depravity of Auschwitz and
other Nazi concentration camps. This, in my opinion, is one of
the greatest books of all time, at the top of my list for inspiring
a renewed sense of purpose and meaning. While sparing the
finer details of Nazi grotesqueness, Frankl describes enough
everyday suffering to make your hair stand on end with his
account of almost unimaginable human cruelty. His humility
and steely resilience in the face of this are an example to
everyone dealing with life's challenges. In his words, 'It did not
really matter what we expected from life, but rather what life

expected from us. Our answer must consist in right action and in right conduct.' One of Frankl's most deeply held values was helping others; throughout his time in the camps, he listened compassionately to the tales of woe of other prisoners, giving words of kindness and inspiration. He consistently tried to support other prisoners to cope with their suffering and tended to the sick and the dying. Most importantly of all, he helped people to connect with their own deepest values so they could find a sense of meaning, which could, quite literally, give them the strength to survive. There are glimpses of awe and hope sprinkled throughout, as Frankl remains calm, composed and compassionate. His willingness at all times to put the needs of others before his own, and his ability to endure, are what set him apart. Perhaps his greatest teaching is that choosing to cultivate purpose and meaning in your life can give you the 'why' to endure any 'how', no matter how severe or arduous. 'When we are no longer able to change a situation, we are challenged to change ourselves.' Despite the harrowing circumstances he found himself in, Frankl understood that he had the power to choose how to respond in any given moment. That in some ways he felt he had more freedom than his Nazi captors, by exercising mindful choice.

A reminder, for me too, of how fortunate I am to live in a place of peace and tranquillity. That peace is a mindful choice, an inner commitment that starts each day in your own heart.

Mindful growth

'*Do not judge me by my successes, judge me by how many times I fell down and got back up again.*'

NELSON MANDELA

N
o one is bulletproof or immune from the flames of burnout. Everyone has some struggles and setbacks in life. Life is rarely plain sailing, for anyone. Some of my challenges have included an arson attack that gutted my first medical premises. The usual degree of swings and roundabouts that come from growing and running a business. Experiencing situational burnout a number of years ago. Challenging times, but in hindsight I am grateful for them, tough and all as they were at the time. I do know that they were mere 'speed bumps' compared with the adversity that many people experience in life. My brush with burnout became my breakthrough to seeing things differently. Taking time to write my *Prescription for Happiness* book became a new starting point for me, reinforcing my view of how resilient I am, helping me to connect with my innate strengths. I reconnected with the essence of who I am, with my purpose of serving others. What's interesting is that once you see things differently, you can never go back to the old way. Once the genie is out of the bottle, there's no putting it

back in! By changing how I saw things, it became a catalyst to gain fresh perspectives, a renewed sense of meaning, to grow.

THE BENEFITS OF RESILIENCE

The philosophy of Navy Seals is a great example of resilience and antifragility. They are able to juggle high levels of operational stress with many competing demands for their attention and focus, while still maintaining a high level of interpersonal functioning. FMRI scans on their brains reveal altered activation in a part of their prefrontal cortex known as the insula, a brain area known to be involved in the management of stress signals.

As a group, Navy Seals exhibit at least seven characteristics of resilient people. These are: calm, innovative, nondogmatic thinking; the ability to act decisively; tenacity; interpersonal connectedness; honesty; self-control; optimism and a positive perspective on life.

In his book *Antifragile: Things That Gain from Disorder*, Nassim Nicholas Taleb defines the term 'antifragile' as describing the person who, just like the Navy Seal, appreciates that stress is part and parcel of life, and that how you respond is what matters most.

I like the term antifragile, which epitomises for me the idea of mindful growth. Being able to embrace stress, strengthen your mindset and gain new perspectives on life's inevitable setbacks and struggles, turning them into opportunities to grow. Understanding that a positive mindset can see more opportunities where the negative mindset simply sees more obstacles.

The acidic soil where I live in Ireland is a happy haven for ericaceous plants like camellias, magnolias and rhododendrons. A few years back, a camellia plant in my garden was really struggling and bedraggled-looking – not a springtime flower in sight. To be honest, I'd completely given up on it and was about to consign it to the compost heap when a friend advised instead to hack it back to just a few inches above the ground and to see what would happen. What wise advice this has turned out to be! Three years later, this plant is sturdy, strong and serenely flourishing. Annual autumn buds signal a forthcoming springtime festival of flowers. A reminder, also, that seeds of growth and green shoots of renewal lie within every dark cloud that appears in your life. If your mind is open to seeing the opportunity for growth, that is!

What does the word 'stress' mean to you in your life? Do you see stress as being harmful or helpful, health-depleting or health-enhancing? Do you believe it should be eradicated or embraced because of its negative or positive effects? If you're like most people, then I can hear your answer loud and clear – because the prevailing mindset is that stress is the silent killer, the all-pervasive destroyer of mental health, physical health and emotional vitality. Indeed, the WHO describes stress as a health epidemic of the twenty-first century, with a wealth of data to highlight the potential impact of toxic stress. In fact, more often than not, rather than wondering *if* stress has played a role, consider just *how much* of a role it plays in most chronic health conditions in the Western world.

Some stress is a fact of life for everyone; part of the living of life itself. What's stressful for one person may not be for another. While you can measure objective levels of stress hormones in research studies, in everyday life it's the degree of stress you feel that's most real.

How do you rate your current stress level on a scale of 1–10 as you are reading this? If you are more than seven, then you are in the red zone. Many people believe they have an unhealthy level of stress in their lives. Doctors have no magic bullet here either; in the medical profession, there are unprecedented levels of professional burnout.

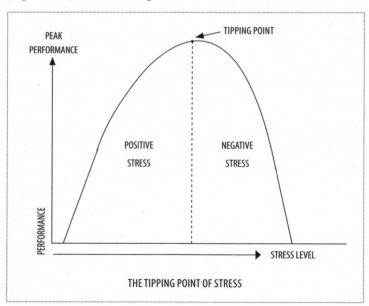

THE TIPPING POINT OF STRESS

The stress response is a key element of survival. However, when this response becomes chronic or prolonged, you pass the tipping point of optimal stress and enter the territory of toxic stress.

THE SCIENCE OF RESILIENCE

When toxic stress builds up, however, it can lead to energy depletion, fatigue and a weakened immune system with increased susceptibility to infection. It results in increased levels of insulin hormone, increased appetite, belly fat storage and cellular inflammation, resulting in increased risk of raised blood pressure, heart disease and diabetes. Toxic stress increases feelings of anxiety, depression and burnout. Stress reduces concentration, memory, productivity and depletes willpower. Chronic toxic stress is corrosive to the brain, damaging the memory centre (hippocampus). The brain becomes more rigid and less malleable (less neuroplasticity) while preventing growth of new brain cells (less neurogenesis).

As the emotional alarm centre (amygdalae) fires at will, it becomes stronger by building new brain connections which take over your hippocampus. This results in memories being branded with fear and toxic stress, which can impact context and perspective and lead to a downward spiral.

However, just as the stress response results in the release of powerful stress hormones like cortisol and adrenaline (as part of the fight, flight or freeze response), it also releases oxytocin, which builds empathy, caring, compassion and the willingness to reach out and connect with others.

Furthermore, recent research from Harvard University has found that oxytocin can heal heart receptors damaged by stress hormones[54]. This acts as a natural counterbalance – a health-boosting yang to the yin of toxic stress. That's the thing about biology and nature. There is an inherent sense of balance and harmony to all things. It is only when you believe the degree of stress is prolonged, and beyond the tipping point, that it becomes a health hazard.

Research in Stanford University has been examining stress-associated mindsets for years. In addition to looking at beliefs about stress, they measure a range of markers from stress hormone levels to how well people manage stress and overall wellbeing[55]. This research has highlighted three interesting findings. Firstly, stress is more likely to be harmful if, because of stress, you experience what I call the 'three Is' of stress – you feel inadequate, invisible or isolated.

Secondly, those people who believe that stress is helpful are more productive and happier at work, less depressed with more confidence to cope with life's challenges. They experience more meaning in the struggles of life and more life satisfaction overall. Thirdly, people who believe stress is helpful have been found to experience just as much stress as those who believe stress is harmful. What's different is their mindset. Perhaps the effect you expect tends to be the effect you get, and that can make all the difference. The key idea is choosing to embrace stress through resilience strategies and restorative recharge rather than simply trying to eradicate stress (which is neither possible nor necessary). In this way, you become more effective at seeing the setbacks and speed bumps that life brings as opportunities to grow and gain new perspectives. Appreciating that you need a certain amount of stress in your life to move forward and perform at your best.

IN MY PRACTICE

Case study time. To the outside world, Conor was the epitome of success, someone who quite literally had it all. A degree in business followed by a prestigious MBA, a successful start-up in Dublin, the new Silicon Valley of Europe. Conor was straight out of the blocks. Now, as a senior executive for a global tech firm, he travelled extensively and his opinions were highly sought after. Married to Katherine with two small children, Conor lived in the affluent leafy suburbs of south county Dublin. He drove a new car, had an exclusive gym membership and, after mortgage and other living expenses, could afford a nice holiday or two each year. On the surface, Conor's life had 'seal of approval' status and appeared to be a recipe for worldly success.

Scratch beneath the surface, though, and cracks were appearing. Always a high achiever at school, some would say Conor was a perfectionist – nothing was ever quite good enough. These perfectionistic traits had followed him his entire life as he climbed the corporate ladders. He was restless, always looking ahead to what was next. He was hard on himself, often pulling 'all-nighters' before tests in college and regularly sacrificing sleep before important assignments in the corporate world. The flip side of this lifestyle and mindset was that Conor was rarely content. He lacked fulfilment and increasingly found himself saying: 'Is this all there is?'

In addition, all that sleep deprivation and the conference calls at crazy hours were taking a toll on his health. He couldn't remember when he had exercised last and had gained about 10 kilograms in weight over the previous two years. His energy was depleted, and he was beginning to feel worn out, at home and at work. In fact, he found that his overall concentration and attention to detail on projects had diminished. As he worked more and more, he got less and less done. When he opened his eyes each morning to a new day, he felt more and more like a cog in an endlessly grinding wheel. His solution of working harder and harder simply wasn't effective any longer. Conor felt increasingly irritable and intolerant. At home, the arguments with Katherine were becoming more frequent and fractious. The spark was gone.

That was the backstory to Conor's life. When he eventually came to see me, he was at breaking point. I hadn't seen Conor for a long time, but he was a long way from the high-energy, bubbly Conor I remembered meeting several years earlier. Years of sacrificing his own self-care had taken their toll and now here he was, sitting in front of me with tears in his eyes. As I listened, he spoke about the sleepless nights and how his sense of self had diminished. How his confidence, self-worth and self-esteem had slowly been eroded away. He had constant feelings of failure and described how he felt crushed. Far from looking forward with confidence to the future, he had a sense of dread. His life was definitely on a downward spiral; he felt weighed down, physically, emotionally and mentally, with nothing left to give. That was it I suppose – more than anything, Conor felt empty.

He needed support to escape those dark days; not just some time out, but a course of medication and talking treatment (counselling) to get back on track. Over time, I worked with Conor, supporting him to make small improvements, step by step, with the focus on progress, not perfection. He learned the benefits of keeping a journal and how expressive writing could allow him to see things differently. He became far more self-aware in terms of how negative thoughts and learned behaviour patterns were holding him back. He became better able to reframe situations in a more positive light, build resilience and a sense of realistic optimism. He also learned the benefits of expressing gratitude as a powerful antidote to feelings of toxic stress and hostility. To be kinder not just to others but also to himself.

Conor set some personal goals for his self-renewal and development as a person. Understanding that actions speak louder than words, he rebuilt positive health habits of restorative sleep, aerobic exercise and good nutrition that aligned with his renewed commitment to his health and vitality. He learned the benefits of mindful meditation: that by creating opportunities for silence and stillness, his authentic inner voice could be heard, and he could tune into who he was and why he mattered.

I recall meeting Conor a few months later and I'm glad to say he really had the courage to walk the walk. In his own words: 'My burnout became my breakthrough to really growing as a person.

I created what I call micro-moments of positivity throughout my day. For example, a short coffee break, stretching my legs with a walk at lunchtime, slowing my breathing for a minute or two. Staying more present. I began to open up, share my story with others and become a better listener. I reduced my exposure to negative noise in the media and in my relationships. More than anything, I realised how priceless health is, and by valuing it through my actions, everyone around me would benefit. I learned that I was responsible for my own choices and that the only person who could make those changes and take back control of my own life was me.'

Conor became emotionally agile, learning to observe his emotions without judgement, the good and the bad. He was able to rebuild a rich emotional bank account of positivity, supporting him to make the best of good times along with the resilience to cope with tough times. Most importantly, Conor learned that he had the ability to grow from his experiences, to choose mindful growth.

THE RESILIENCE PRESCRIPTION

I believe **resilience** starts the moment you acknowledge and accept the reality you find yourself in. Facing and embracing adversity leads to growth. Denying, or suppressing it emotionally, simply leads to more suffering. **Acceptance** of what you can and can't control is so liberating and emotionally freeing. Acceptance becomes the new starting point from which to move forward, one choice, one step, one day at a time. It is a mindset change from scarcity to abundance, from 'what I have lost' to 'how can I grow?'

Recharging from stress is your responsibility. In other words, your response to and ability to regularly recharge is the key to preventing the adverse effects of toxic stress. Instead of trying to eradicate stress, learn more skills to embrace stress. Here are some strategies to help you in this practice:

Recognise your stress mindset: Understand that stress in and of itself is neither good nor bad. How do you see stress? – as something harmful or helpful?

Reframe: Keeping a written journal can enable you to reframe experiences, setbacks and adversity through the lens of growth, meaning and connection. Growth comes not from trauma itself (which of course is inherently bad), but from the response to the trauma in terms of becoming stronger, kinder and more resilient. Ask yourself: what can you learn from this situation? How can you use this experience as an opportunity to grow?

Philosophers of old used three separate lenses through which to examine an experience: Firstly, the **long lens**: Will this issue I'm concerned about still matter a year from now? If not, why am I giving it so much attention? Secondly, the **reverse lens**: How might this issue look from the other person's perspective? In what aspects might they be right? Thirdly, the **wide lens**: Things happen in life that I can't change or control. How then can this experience become an opportunity to learn and grow?

Mindful choice: Choosing to focus more of your attentive awareness on those things you can control, and the positive actions you can take, is empowering and builds autonomy – a key variable in wellbeing. In other words, focusing on the circle of control as opposed to the circle of concern.

Mindful optimism: Researchers asked people in the USA, India and Canada if they believed life to be long or short, easy or hard. The majority considered life to be short and hard, with barely one in eight considering life to be long and easy. These were the optimists, who were found to be significantly happier as well as more likely to give to charity, to vote and to volunteer in their local community. The mindful optimist is someone who embraces stress, experiences setbacks and uses them as an opportunity to grow and to learn. The mindful optimist is resilient, gritty and never stops starting. The mindful optimist doesn't believe in fairy tales, grounding their optimistic worldview in their own efforts. I call mindful optimism the 'oxygen for opportunity' in life. Of course, mindful or realistic optimism is the belief that things can get better because you are going to do something about it – your everyday choice to see the glass as half-full rather than half-empty, to turn your stumbling blocks into stepping-stones of opportunity. Mindful optimism comes in part from your generalised expectations for a good outcome (known as dispositional optimism), in addition to how you interpret and explain good and bad news. The key difference between the optimist and the pessimist is that the optimist sees life's challenges as being temporary, controllable and specific to one situation. More importantly, the optimist doesn't take it personally.

The pessimist will assume the three P's:

O   Personalised – 'It's my fault.'

O   Pervasive (generalised) – 'This impacts everything.'

O   Permanent – 'It will last forever.'

The mindful optimist is better able to downplay negative thoughts and feelings, to adopt a better coping style. To plan, persevere and become more resilient. While understanding that setbacks are an inevitable part of life, the mindful optimist becomes more effective at navigating those setbacks as opportunities to grow and to ultimately become stronger. Seeing the world through the lens of mindful optimism can support your physical health with a stronger immune system. You are more likely to report feeling better with higher subjective wellbeing than equally healthy people who are pessimistic. Why optimism is so beneficial for your vitality remains unclear. Perhaps due to lower levels of stress hormones and inflammatory markers or perhaps due in part to healthier lifestyles or stronger support networks. Mindful optimism can significantly reduce your risk of heart disease, stroke or death from cardiovascular causes, in fact by up to 35 per cent according to the *Journal of the American Medical Association*. On the other hand, pessimism can be very bad for both your blood pressure and heart health. The Nurses' Health Study, which has been following the health and health-related behaviours of a large group of American nurses since 1976, has found a strong and statistically significant association between raised levels of optimism and reduced mortality.

In terms of your mental health, mindful optimists tend to experience less stress, anxiety and depression. By learning to reframe challenging situations in a more positive way, you dissipate toxic stress and tend to handle stressful situations better. More effective coping strategies help tip the scales of positivity back in your direction. Mindful optimism can sometimes protect you from accurately seeing the pain and challenges that the future may hold, which can be a good thing, at times. Overall, you become grittier and more resilient, better able to deal with setbacks and ultimately more successful.

Emotionally, optimism supports a stronger sense of hope, with more confidence, positivity and willingness to believe it is possible. You tend to be more positive, energised and happier, with more friends and stronger interpersonal relationships.

Remember self-care: Unfortunately, self-care is often one of the first casualties of toxic stress. People can retreat into their shell and stop taking good care of themselves at a time when they need self-care more than ever. Furthermore, stress depletes willpower, bringing forth self-destructive habits, behaviours and unhealthy coping strategies that may feel good in the moment but are the antithesis of self-care. Investing in your own self-care means including physical, psychological, emotional and spiritual aspects on an ongoing basis. I believe in prescribing a strategy of self-care – I call it radical self-care – because it really is that important.

In Japanese culture, the presence of the flaw intensifies and deepens the degree of an object's beauty. Every work of art has a flaw and one rarely meets an artist entirely happy with their work. As the saying goes, there is a flaw of imperfection in every sparkling diamond. *Wabi-sabi* is a Zen concept of showcasing flaws as something beautiful that personalise and enhance rather than detract from an object's value. For example, the asymmetry of the drawing, a blemish in the painting or crack in the vase. The inherent beauty in that which is impermanent, incomplete and imperfect – but, above all, authentic and real.

Kintsugi is the Japanese tradition of repairing cracked pottery. Instead of trying to camouflage the cracks, the broken pieces of pottery are repaired using a lacquer mixed with powdered aluminium, silver or gold. The finished product is pottery that looks beautiful because of, rather than in spite of, its brokenness. For me, the wisdom of wabi-sabi and kintsugi are wonderful metaphors for the tremendous capacity of human beings to transcend setbacks and struggles in a way that leads to post-traumatic growth. A flaw can be a destructive, damaging and diminishing force, or it can be integrated and offer you freedom. You see the world less as it is, and more as you are. Neuroscience backs this up, with recent research showing that at least 80 per cent of what you see is based on your brain's interpretation of reality. If you focus on your flaws and imperfections, they can feel like a weight holding you back. By changing the way you look at things, the things you look at can start to change. So don't let your flaws, weaknesses or imperfections weigh you down in the sea of life. Choose to see your flaws for what they really are: the opportunity to accept the fullness of who you are. As an opportunity to grow and shine brightly in the world. To embrace a more genuine and authentic version of you: imperfect, flawed and still a wonderful human being.

Your future self: Imagine a time in the future – say five years from now – when you have realised your potential and everything you have worked towards comes to pass. This is not a delusional dream: it's deliberately mapping out your future based on efforts that are realistic, positive and achievable. Visualise this future clearly in all the various domains of your life. Write it down on paper in terms of your relationships, health, career and self-development. Include places you hope to travel to, hobbies you want to learn, books you want to read. Imagine working hard to realise your potential. Writing your best possible future down on paper gives it granular clarity and makes it more real. How does this 'future self' look like to you? How will it feel to achieve these goals? This exercise is a terrific way to build positive emotion, strengthen mindful optimism and support you in living with more vitality. As Swami Vivekananda wrote: 'We are responsible for what we are, and whatever we wish ourselves to be, we have the power to make ourselves'.

Write to grow: One of the best ways to support post-traumatic growth is through expressive writing. This has been described eloquently by Professor James Pennebaker at the University of Texas, based on his own life experiences. In the early years of his marriage, his relationship with his spouse was struggling, and his life spiralled downwards into depression. One day he got out of bed and began to write freely about his life and all his issues. He continued this day after day, and began to notice that he felt better. Not only did his depression lift, but he was able to rebuild his relationship with his wife and reframe his life overall through the lens of purpose. This personal growth became his catalyst for a fascinating career researching the benefits of expressive writing. In summary, he has found benefits from simply writing about an issue of concern or worry for a period of about 15 minutes each day for three consecutive days. After this time period, you can tear up what you've written. You don't need to write perfect prose, a stream of consciousness will do just fine. This expressive writing has been subjected to hundreds of research studies which have found numerous benefits. It can ease feelings of anxiety and depression, boost sleep, support the immune system, build resilience and interpersonal relationships. Overall, it supports enhanced overall wellbeing and vitality. Furthermore, expressive writing has been shown to support growth from a range of traumatic life events. Pennebaker's research on middle-aged men who lost their engineering jobs after a company downsizing found they were three times more likely to be re-employed elsewhere within six months if they did the expressive writing exercise (and wrote about their feelings of losing their job, rejection, etc.). His career and longstanding research have shown conclusively that writing about your emotional experiences is extremely beneficial for your health and wellbeing. It appears that the act of writing forces the mind to slow down, to become more intentional, to make sense of ruminative thoughts, and to create meaning and patterns between previous and current events. Writing also encourages you to ask important questions, including why did this happen, what does it mean and what happens next? It also creates a sense of separation from the event or experience you are writing about which in itself can create the space for new perspectives. Writing through this lens can enable you to see things differently and change the dialogue from how you have suffered to how you can grow. Expressive writing can allow you to become the hero in your own story, as you reframe from 'I am a victim' to 'I am a survivor'. This can lead to a fundamental shift in sense of self in terms of enhancing self-improvement. You learn to place more emphasis on the present moment as opposed to the pain of the past. As you also become more forward-looking and more of a mindful optimist, you build resilience to future stressors.

Many people experience positive growth in the aftermath of stressful setbacks and adversity. The National Institute of Mental Health in the US has highlighted that while more than 50 per cent of people experience at least one traumatic event in their lifetime (loss, bereavement, serious illness, displacement, war, famine, natural disasters, unemployment or relationship issues), the majority do not develop post-traumatic stress. By contrast, many grow in time from their experience – welcome to the idea of post-traumatic growth.

Research from Stanford University highlights that one of

the most common effects of stress is growth or resilience[56]. Areas where growth may occur include spiritual change, change in use of personal strengths (especially gratitude, resilience and optimism), more appreciation of life and those people that matter, improved relationships with others, enhanced compassion and altruism, and new perspectives on life itself in terms of how to live, sense of purpose and relationships.

In summary, stress can become a physical, mental and emotional health hazard, or stress can become a catalyst for growth and resilience. As well as learning to recharge from stress, the challenge is to develop the self-awareness to reframe your mindset to see stress as something to embrace, something that can support you in becoming wiser, stronger and better.

You live in a world of instant gratification and the quick fix. In healthcare, this can manifest as the pill for every ill, the sticking plaster solution; in the media, the sound bites and never-ending promises. However, there is no shortcut to mindful growth or wisdom. There is no substitute for long-term thinking, for deep learning, where knowledge turns to wisdom through the application of learned experience.

While achievements gather dust in the memories of your past, and shiny goals can illuminate your future, they are never destinations, simply markers along the path. A commitment to practise is a present-moment activity. Something to experience and embrace in the present moment.

Journal

Take some time to reflect on this last set of journaling questions, trying to draw on everything we have covered in this section so far:

Think of a time when you experienced a stressful event, something that mattered to you, a relationship or health issue, job interview, etc.

O   How did you deal with this at the time?

O   How did you react or respond?

Now reassess the situation from the perspective of growth.

O   What did you learn from this experience?

O   How have you grown as a result?

Spend a few minutes describing this experience through the following areas:

O   Spiritual growth

O   Personal strength

O   Appreciation for life

O   Increased social connections and interpersonal relationships

O   New possibilities and life directions.

The path of progress is a journey, enabling often invisible progress along a never-ending plateau. Just like the camellia plant, perhaps the struggles from life's everyday stresses can support you to grow, gain new perspectives, reach your full potential and experience mindful growth. The joy of the journey is the journey itself, the commitment to consistency and progress. To never stop learning and growing. To live with more vitality.

CONCLUSION

Vitality – a new vital sign

'*We shall not cease from exploration, and the end of all our exploring will be to arrive where we started and know the place for the first time.*'

T.S. ELIOT

Having been born in January, I've always had a special affiliation with this month, despite its association in Ireland with wintry weather. The word 'January' originated from the Roman God Janus – symbolising doorways, and new beginnings. While often depicted as having two heads, my favourite representation of Janus actually has three heads that simultaneously look back at the past, straight ahead and forward into the future. A terrific reminder of the potential we all have to learn from the past, to live in the present while looking forward with optimism and vitality to a brighter future.

If you have got to this page of the book, then congratulations. You have come a long way! By investing your time (hopefully enjoyably), I hope this book has given you some ideas and strategies to enable you to live with more vitality.

Has it? What might you now see differently in terms of your vitality? What are your personal insights, reflections and learnings? It's so easy to forget key ideas once a book is finished. More often than not, people simply move on. Taking some time to write down the strategies learned can deepen the learning. Use the table format below to consolidate what you have learned.

New insight	Why is this important to you?	How can you apply it in your life?
Gratitude		
Kindfulness		
Negativity		
Sleep		
Movement		
Eating		
Purpose		
Meditation		
Nature		
Mindful presence		
Mindful choice		
Mindful growth		

None of us can go back to the beginning and start again, but starting today, you can create a brand-new narrative in your life. My question for you is: how can you close your intention gap to move closer to your best self and live with more vitality? I encourage you to not just read but reread, highlight and underscore those ideas that are most relevant to you. Deepen and internalise those ideas that matter. Own them. Make them real.

Mandala as a word comes from the ancient Sanskrit language. While literally speaking it means circle, or wholeness, it is seen in all cultures and religions. Buddhist monks can spend many hours, even days, handcrafting their beautiful mandalas entirely from sand. The construction of these intricate geometric designs requires intense concentration and is itself a form of meditative practice, creating an awareness of being part of something bigger than your own world. Once completed, the monks pray over the finished mandala and then promptly destroy it, shattering any illusions of attachment and permanency. Some handfuls of sand may be given to participants in the closing ceremony as a token of possibility, while the rest is thrown into a nearby stream to be swept away and to bless the entire world. The mandala symbolises the impermanence and transitory nature of the material world.

The Buddhist mandala is an interesting way to approach everything in life. You build things, they break down. You clean your kitchen, it becomes untidy again. In this way, life becomes an unending, ephemeral process of continuous change and new beginnings. Understanding this mindful truth is a key to wisdom. The idea is to never stop starting: the only constant is constant change. You may learn something, try it out and step forward, then slip back. That's okay. It's all about progress. Simply start again.

I love the definition of health as 'the crown on the well person's head that only the sick person may see'. We can all be guilty of taking good health for granted, unless or until something happens, and you may spend every minute scrambling to get your health back. If you believe, as I do, that your health is a priceless asset, then living with vitality becomes a new commitment to lead your own life in terms of your everyday choices and commitments.

To become an active participant in your own wellbeing, rather than a passive consumer of healthcare. To listen to your heart, live by your values and let your lifestyle become your best possible medicine. To understand that self-care is the foundation stone for you and everyone that matters in your life. To embrace the uniqueness of who you are – the good, the not-so-good and the beauty of your imperfections.

To accept your flaws, let go of the pain of perfectionism and embrace the wisdom of wabi-sabi. To acknowledge just how far you have come already in your life; the hurdles overcome, the small victories, the courage you have shown. To accept that setbacks, struggles and stressful times are all part of life's journey. To accept that mistakes are part and parcel of being human, to gift yourself forgiveness and move on. That an immutable truth is that the seeds of good fortune lie within bad fortune and vice versa, that success and failure are two sides of the same coin. To face your fears, follow your heart and find your flow. To embrace change. To stay open, in your heart and mind, to opportunity and possibility. To stay in touch with the timeless wisdom of the *Tao Te Ching*, by embracing simplicity, compassion and humility. To choose kindness and an attitude of gratitude and appreciation.

Above all, to remember that you have the power to choose how to respond in any given moment. To choose more wisely and not become a victim of toxic stress or reactive circumstance. To live with purpose, in alignment with your strengths and values. To adopt a mindset of growth, in seeing your life through the lens of experience, moving from what you have lost to how you can grow. To take good care of your body, your mind, your heart and your spirit. To make time for those people and things that matter most. To laugh, lighten up, remain true to yourself, authentic, vulnerable and real. To have an inner knowing that your vitality is in you and it is you. To stay in tune with it and leverage it for your benefit. To never stop learning and growing. To never stop starting.

To your vitality.

Endnotes

1 Herskind A.M. et al. (1996). The heritability of human longevity: a population-based study of 2872 Danish twin pairs born 1870-1900. *Human Genetics*, 97 (3), 319-23.

2 Li, Y., Schoufour, J., Wang, D.D., Dhana, K., Pan, A., Liu, X. et al. (2020). Healthy lifestyle and life expectancy free of cancer, cardiovascular disease, and type 2 diabetes: prospective cohort study. *BMJ*.

3 Levy, B.R., Slade, M.D., Kunkel, S.R., & Kasl, S.V. (2002). Longevity increased by positive self-perceptions of aging. *Journal of Personality and Social Psychology*, 83 (2), 261–270.

4 Miller, W.R. & Rollnick, S. (2013). *Motivational Interviewing: Helping People Change*. (New York, NY: Guilford Press.)

5 (1940). NORTHERN THEATRE: Sisu. www.TIME.com.

6 Lally, P., van Jaarsveld, C.H.M., Potts, H.W.W., & Wardle, J. (2009). How are habits formed: Modelling habit formation in the real world. *European Journal of Social Psychology*.

7 Davidson, R.J. (2008). Buddha's brain: neuroplasticity and meditation. *IEEE Signal Processing Magazine*, 25 (1), 176–174.

8 Emmons, R.A., & Mishra, A. (2011). Why gratitude enhances well-being: What we know, what we need to know. In K.M. Sheldon, T.B. Kashdan, & M.F. Steger (Eds.), *Designing positive psychology: Taking stock and moving forward* (pp. 248–262). Oxford University Press.

9 Emmons, R.A. (2008). *Thanks! How Practicing Gratitude Can Make You Happier* (1st ed.). HarperOne.

10 Fox, G. R. (2015). *Neural correlates of gratitude*. Frontiers in Psychology.

11 Alkozei, A., Smith, R., & Killgore, W. D. (2018). *Gratitude and subjective wellbeing: A proposal of two causal frameworks*. Journal of Happiness Studies, 19: 1519–1542.

12 Emmons, R.A. (2008).

13 Rakel, D.P. et al. (2009). Practitioner empathy and the duration of the common cold. *Family Medicine*, 41 (7), 494–501.

14 Trew, J.L. & Alden, L.E. (2015). Kindness reduces avoidance goals in socially anxious individuals. *Motivation and Emotion*, 39 (6), 892–907.

15 Zaki, J. (2016). Kindness Contagion. *Scientific American*. https://www.scientificamerican.com/article/kindness-contagion/

16 Lyubomirsky, Sonja. (2010). *The How of Happiness*. Piatkus Books.

17 Small acts of kindness at work benefit the giver, the receiver and the whole organisation. (2017). *Research Digest*.

18 Le Nguyen, K.D., Fredrickson, B.L. et al. (2009). Loving-kindness meditation slows biological aging in novices: Evidence from a 12-week randomized controlled trial. *Psychoneuroendocrinology*, 108, 20–27.

19 Cacioppo J.T., Cacioppo S., Gollan J.K. (2014). The negativity bias: Conceptualization, quantification, and individual differences. *Behavioral and Brain Sciences*, 37 (3), 309–310.

20 Sleep-Related Behaviors – 12 States, 2009. (2011). www.cdc.gov.

21 Hanlon, E.C. et al. (2016). Sleep restriction enhances the daily rhythm of circulating levels of endocannabinoid 2-arachidonoylglycerol. *Sleep*, 39 (3), 653–664.

22 van der Ploeg, H.P., Chey, T., Korda, R.J., Banks, E. & Bauman, A. (2012). Sitting time and all-cause mortality risk in 222,497 Australian adults. *Archives of Internal Medicine*, 172 (6), 494–500.

23 Nam, J.Y., Kim, J., Cho, K.H. et al. (2017). The impact of sitting time and physical activity on major depressive disorder in South Korean adults: a cross-sectional study. *BMC Psychiatry* 17, 274.

24 Cuthbertson, C.C., Tan, X., et al. (2019). Associations of leisure-time physical activity and television viewing with life expectancy free of non-fatal cardiovascular disease: the ARIC study. *Journal of the American Heart Association*, 8 (18).

25 Oaten, M. & Cheng, K. (2006). Longitudinal gains in self-regulation from regular physical exercise. *Br J Health Psychol*. 11 (4), 717-33.

26 Puterman, E., Lin, J. et al. (2010). The power of exercise: buffering the effect of chronic stress on telomere length. *PLoS One*, 5 (5).

27 Zhang, Z., Chen, W. (2019). A systematic review of the relationship between physical activity and happiness. *Journal of Happiness Studies*, 20, 1305–1322.

28 Wiedemann, K., Jahn, H., Yassouridis, A. & Kellner, M. (2001). Anxiolytic-like effects of atrial natriuretic peptide on cholecystokinin tetrapeptide-induced panic attacks: preliminary findings. *Archives of General Psychiatry*, 58 (4), 371–377.

29 Martínez-González, M.A., Gea, A., & Ruiz-Canela, M. (2019). The Mediterranean diet and cardiovascular health. *Circulation Research*, 124 (5), 779–798.

30 Paterson, K.E., Myint, P.K. et al. (2018). Mediterranean diet reduces risk of incident stroke in a population with varying cardiovascular disease risk profiles. *Stroke*, 49: 2415–2420.

31 Yong, E. (2014). How jetlag disrupts the ticks of your microbial clock. *National Geographic*.

32 Wilkinson, M. J., Manoogian, E. N. C. et al. (2020). Ten-hour time-restricted eating reduces weight, blood pressure, and atherogenic lipids in patients with metabolic syndrome. *Cell Metabolism*, 31 (1), 92–104.

33 Sone, T., Nakaya, N., Ohmori, K. et al. (2008). Sense of life worth living (*ikigai*) and mortality in Japan: Ohsaki study. *Psychosomatic Medicine*, 70 (6), 709–15.

34 Tang, Y., Lu, Q., Posner, M. et al. (2010). Short-term meditation induces white matter changes in the anterior cingulate. *Proceedings of the National Academy of Sciences*.

35 Lazar, S.W., Kerr, C.E., Wasserman, R.H., et al. (2005). Meditation experience is associated with increased cortical thickness. *Neuroreport*, 16 (17), 1893–1897.

36 Fox K.C., Nijeboer S., Dixon M.L., et al. (2014). Is meditation associated with altered brain structure? A systematic review and meta-analysis of morphometric neuroimaging in meditation practitioners. *Neuroscience & Biobehavioral Reviews*, 43, 48-73.

37 Bratman, G.N., et al. (2015). Nature reduces rumination and subgenual prefrontal cortex activation. *Proceedings of the National Academy of Sciences*, 112 (28), 8567-8572

38   Kim, G.W., et al. (2010). Functional neuroanatomy associated with natural and urban scenic views in the human brain: 3.0T Functional MR Imaging. *Korean Journal of Radiology*, 11 (5), 507-513.

39   Engemann, K. et al. (2019). Residential green space in childhood is associated with lower risk of psychiatric disorders from adolescence into adulthood. *Proceedings of the National Academy of Sciences*, 116 (11), 5188-5193.

40   Williams, K. & L., et al. (2018). Conceptualising creativity benefits of nature experience: Attention restoration and mind wandering as complementary processes. *Journal of Environmental Psychology*, 59.

41   Stellar J.E. et al. (2015). Positive affect and markers of inflammation: discrete positive emotions predict lower levels of inflammatory cytokines. *Emotion*, 15 (2), 129-33.

42   Ochiai, H., Ikei, H., et al. (2015). Physiological and psychological effects of forest therapy on middle-aged males with high-normal blood pressure. *International journal of environmental research and public health*, 12 (3), 2532–2542.

43   Lichtenfeld, S., Elliot, A. J., Maier, M. A. & Pekrun, R. (2012). Fertile green: green facilitates creative performance. *Personality and Social Psychology Bulletin*, 38(6): 784–797.

44   Nass, C. et al. (2009). Cognitive control in media multitaskers. *Proceedings of the National Academy of Sciences*, 106 (37) 15583-15587.

45   Tseng, J., Poppenk, J. (2020). Brain meta-state transitions demarcate thoughts across task contexts exposing the mental noise of trait neuroticism. *Nature Communications*, 11, 3480.

46   Shaner, L., Kelly, L., Rockwell, D., & Curtis, D. (2016). Calm abiding. *Journal of Humanistic Psychology*, 57 (1), 98–121.

47   Taren, A.A. et al. (2015). Mindfulness meditation training alters stress-related amygdala resting state functional connectivity: a randomized controlled trial. *Social cognitive and affective neuroscience*, 10(12), 1758–1768.

48   Kirste, I., et al. (2015). Is silence golden? Effects of auditory stimuli and their absence on adult hippocampal neurogenesis. *Brain structure & function*, 220 (2), 1221–1228.

49   McMains, S. & Kastner, S. (2011). Interactions of top-down and bottom-up mechanisms in human visual cortex. *Journal of Neuroscience*, 31 (2) 587-597.

50   Steffen, P.R., Austin, T., DeBarros, A., & Brown, T. (2017). The impact of resonance frequency breathing on measures of heart rate variability, blood pressure, and mood. *Frontiers in Public Health*, 5, 222.

51   Hanley, A.W., Warner, A.R., Dehili, V.M. et al. (2015). Washing dishes to wash the dishes: brief instruction in an informal mindfulness practice. *Mindfulness* 6, 1095–1103.

52   Gable, S.L., Reis, H.T., Impett, E.A., & Asher, E.R. (2004). What do you do when things go right? The intrapersonal and interpersonal benefits of sharing positive events. *Journal of Personality and Social Psychology*, 87 (2), 228–245.

53   McGonigal, K. (2016). *The Upside of Stress: Why Stress Is Good for You, and How to Get Good at It* (Reprint ed.). Avery.

54   Jankowski, M., Broderick, T.L., & Gutkowska, J. (2020). The Role of Oxytocin in Cardiovascular Protection. *Frontiers in Psychology*, 11, 2139.

55   McGonigal, K.

56   McGonigal, K.